PERCEPTIONS AND REPRESENTATIONS

The theoretical bases of brain research and psychology

Perceptions and Representations

THE THEORETICAL BASES OF BRAIN RESEARCH AND PSYCHOLOGY

KEITH OATLEY

METHUEN & CO LTD

First published in 1978
by Methuen & Co Ltd
11 New Fetter Lane, London EC4P 4EE

Typeset by Red Lion Setters
and printed in Great Britain
at the University Printing House,
Cambridge

ISBN 0 416 86010 9

Contents

To
Simon
and
Grant

Preface

This book is largely about perception. In it I try to give a percept of physiological psychology, experimental psychology and neurophysiology as activities which are, in part, misdirected. The percept is a view from one side of a Kuhnian paradigm gap, and the side is the opposite one to that adopted in most physiological psychology texts.

This percept is like one view of an ambiguous figure. It does not deny the existence of the other view, rather as this view is invoked the other one is lost, momentarily or perhaps for longer. To use a somewhat sexist image, it is as if in Boring's wife/mistress figure I try to articulate first the somewhat unprepossessing features of the older lady, and then later in the book the more seductive ones of the younger lady. But perhaps as the new paradigm arises it may be possible to transcend the mutual incompatibility of the two views. In this way, in science, if not in the perception of ambiguous figures, we perhaps need not forever flip between two incompatible views.

I feel also that I should declare at least some of my biases. I see myself as having taken part, in research and teaching, in many of the activities of neurophysiology, experimental and physiological psychology described here; and grown through them and out of them. From this stance I can take a certain emotional satisfaction in being somewhat rejecting.

The first eight chapters contain discussions of some implications of seeing the brain as conferring meaning on the data arising from the world, and arguments for seeing mental processes not in terms of analysing stimuli, but in terms of mental representations and schemata. The last chapter suggests a further shift of paradigm towards a psychology seeking not just for explanations, but insights into our mental life.

In the writing of this book I owe debts of gratitude to a large number of people. When the book was started many years ago it was to have been a text in physiological psychology. It has changed fundamentally since then, and not least I am grateful to the publishers, who have put up with my temporizations. I am grateful to students, teachers and colleagues too numerous to mention who have helped in many ways in the shaping of my thoughts. In particular, I would like to thank Max Clowes who introduced me to artificial intelligence. Most of all, I would like to thank the people who have typed and helped in the production of various drafts: Amanda Cooper, Anne Doidge, Stella Frost, Sheila Lawrence and Monica Robinson.

Acknowledgments

The author and publishers would like to thank the following for permission to reproduce the copyright material which appears in this book:

James MacGibbon for the poem 'Not Waving But Drowning' in *The Collected Poems of Stevie Smith*; Professor N.S. Sutherland for Table 1; G. Johansson and the University of Uppsala for Fig. 1.2; D.B. Burns for Fig. 3.1a; Cambridge University Press for Fig. 3.2; American Association for the Advancement of Science for Fig. 4.3; Williams & Williams Co. for Fig. 4.5; Harcourt, Brace and World for Fig. 5.1; Pergamon Press for Fig. 5.3; Professor M.B. Clowes for Fig. 7.2; Massachusetts Institute of Technology for Figs 7.3 and 7.5; Karl Dallenbach for Figs 7.6 and 8.3; Dr. P. Lennie for Fig. 8.1; Optical Society of America for Fig. 8.2; M.L.J. Abercrombie for Fig. 8.4; Academic Press for Figs 8.5 and 8.6; North Holland Publishing Co. for Figs 8.7 and 8.10.

And when a book's pattern and the shape of its inner life is as plain to the reader as it is to the author — then perhaps it is time to throw the book aside, as having had its day, and start again on something new.

Doris Lessing, 1971, from the preface to *The Golden Notebook*

1 *Lashley and some fundamental problems in psychology*

The three themes of this book are the relation of the brain's structure to psychological function, the problem of how people perceive successfully in a world where evidence presented to the senses is rather degenerate and fragmentary, and the role of theory in understanding neural and mental processes.

We live in a world in which we perceive objects fulfilling particular functions that serve our purposes. A chair, for instance, is easily recognizable. It is an artificial, solid object in the outside world with a surface raised above the ground, and suitable for supporting the human bottom. It has a back against which a person's back can rest while he or she is sitting. But a chair which we might see is also a mental construct: it is a mental representation of an object capable of supporting the sitting body.

Although phenomenally we seem to be able to experience such objects in the outside world with immediacy, we do not 'sense' them directly. We experience them via the mental representations we have of them. Expanding on this notion, it is possible to show that the world contains an indefinitely large number of objects which we would recognize as chairs, yet they are either in detail or in gross appearance different from one another. Furthermore, we can recognize chairs from an indefinitely large number of viewpoints, in an indefinitely large number of contexts, and with a very substantial degree of occlusion of the chair from our viewpoint. In fig. 1.1, for instance, we have no difficulty in recognizing a curved dark area which indicates the existence of a chair in this scene. Putting it another way, what is presented to our sensory receptors is fragmentary, and very different from the interpretations which constitute our experience and which are in terms not of signals from the retina, or fragments of lines, but in terms of solid objects in the world. No finite set of retinal patterns would specify the class of chairs, yet with a finite brain we do see definite chairs.

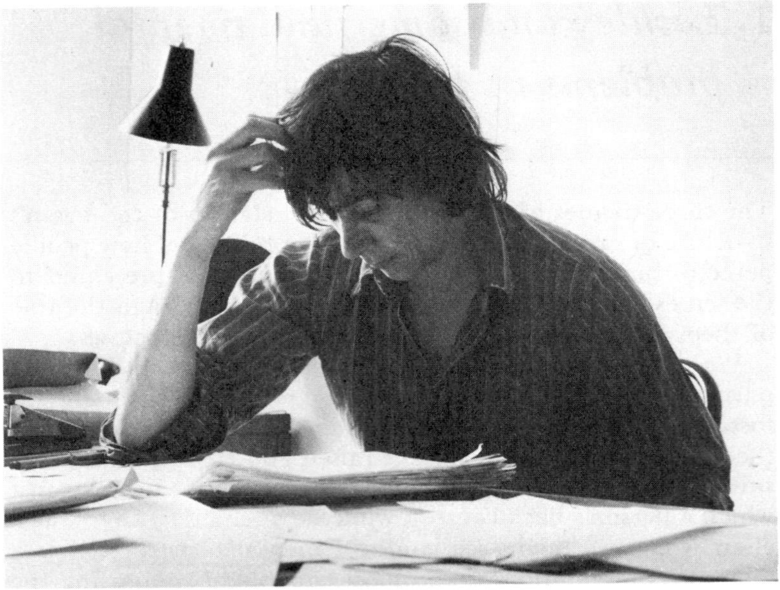

Figure 1.1 Fragmentary evidence and context allow us to recognise a chair in this scene.

This kind of puzzling difference between what seems to be the domain of our retinal images and the world of our mental awareness may make one wonder whether ideas are more real than the sensory appearances of the material world. These sensory appearances are at best degenerate facsimiles of reality. Certainly any particular retinal image of a chair from a particular viewpoint is for us a degenerate facsimile, a fleeting two-dimensional projection on the retina of a three-dimensional object. Yet our perception of a particular chair is not of the chair's image, but of the chair, and is such that we know a great deal about it, whether it would be comfortable, hard or soft, cheap or expensive, what it would look like from the other side and so on.

Plato in book VII of *The Republic* (e.g. edited by Hamilton and Cairns, 1961) has a simile of man's predicament. Living consciously in a world of ideas yet physically in a world of appearances, people are like men in a cave; fettered with their eyes looking at one wall, and with their backs to a fire which casts shadows of themselves and of various objects on the wall in front of them. They might see 'men carrying past the wall implements of all kinds ... and human images and shapes of animals as well'. The point Plato wanted to make from this was that the men in the cave think the shadows (which correspond to the degenerate appearances in the physical world) are reality. In Plato's simile people have to become freed of their fetters, constraining them to look at the shadows, and force their minds to the bright but painful glare of light at the cave's entrance and make a long difficult journey upwards and out of the cave to the daylight where they can see the real world.

However, the story could go another way. The shadows are like the patterns falling on our receptors. But with a theory of the process of casting shadows, and knowledge of the kinds of objects that could be casting the shadows, we can understand from the distorted and flickering phantoms of shadow what is going on in the middle world of people between the fire and the shadows. Our ideas, or interpretations, guided by the theory of shadow casting, bring us into touch with a reality, indeed closer to a reality, of more practical use to us than the shadows. When conducting ourselves in the world we do not see the flickering shadows on our retina. We actually see our interpretations of what is happening in the world, people, objects, fields, trees and so on, disposed in three-dimensional space. Any demonstration, such as fig. 1.1, indeed a glance around a room where many objects will be partly obscured and all seen from only one direction, will illustrate this. Incomplete figures or cartoons are not as special as they may seem; they merely demonstrate the ability of our minds to cope with fragmentariness. Some of the best demonstrations of this are kinetic ones, such as those of Johansson (1971) of which a single still picture appears in fig. 1.2a. The spots of light which are all that appear on a film which Johansson has made are in fact carried by a person as in fig. 1.2b, and on watching a moving film of just the spots one sees not just moving spots. One recognizes a person, with an almost perceptible shadowy body and limbs performing easily recognizable movements of walking, dancing, etc.

An important fact about visual images (retinal or otherwise) is that such appearances are fragmentary (maximally from one viewpoint we can only see one side of an object), yet we experience a very solid complete world. This book is about the question of what processes or mechanisms could be capable of

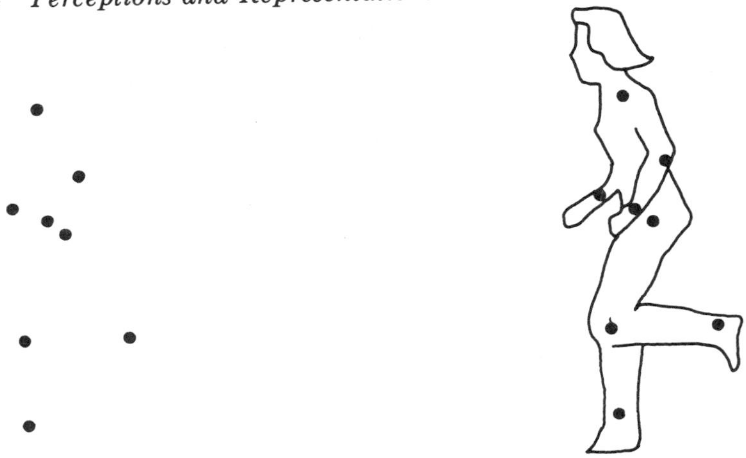

a b

Figure 1.2 The pattern of dots in (a) is unrecognisable, but when they move, the outline of a person is projected or hallucinated as in (b), (redrawn from Johansson 1971).

mediating between the shadows that fall on our sense organs and the conscious experience of meaningful reality which we believe we have. How can neural structure subserve this function? What kinds of theories in psychology illuminate the issue of how the brain can perform this type of function, and what organizations of process can begin to achieve interpretations of fragmentary flickering shadows?

Some of the inspiration for this book comes from the work of Karl Lashley. He might be argued to be the founder of physiological psychology. He identified some crucial issues in that subject, and, in particular, the following: the relation of structure to function, the problem of fragmentariness and inconstancy of sensory input, and the issue of how theories of brains illuminate the difficult problem of understanding the mind. These three issues are rather aptly illustrated by three quotations from Lashley.

(1) Most of our (psychology) textbooks begin with an exposition of the structure of the brain, and imply that this lays a foundation for a later understanding of behaviour ... The chapter on the nervous system seems to provide an

excuse for pictures in an otherwise dry and monotonous text. That it has any other function is not clear. (1930)

(2) Here is the dilemma. Nerve impulses are transmitted over definite restricted paths ... yet all behaviour seems to be determined by masses of excitation, by the form or relations or proportions of excitation within general fields of activity without regard to particular nerve cells. It is the pattern and not the element that counts. (1942)

(3) I am less impressed with the analogies between various machines and neural activity, such as are discussed in Cybernetics. There has been a curious parallel in the histories of neurological theories and of paranoid delusional systems. In Mesmer's day the paranoid was persecuted by malicious animal magnetism, his successors by galvanic shocks, by the telegraph, by radio, and by radar, keeping their delusional systems up to date with the latest fashions in physics. Descartes was impressed by the hydraulic figures in the royal gardens and developed a hydraulic theory of the action of the brain. We have since had telephone theories, electrical field theories, and now theories based on the computing machines and automatic rudders. I suggest that we are more likely to find out how the brain works by studying the brain itself and the phenomena of behaviour than by indulging in far-fetched physical analogies. The similarities in such comparisons are the product of an oversimplification of the problems of behaviour ... (1951)

Given these three quotations I follow some of Lashley's recommendations. There is no chapter on the structure of the nervous system. But this book does contain some discussion of how far anatomy and related studies are important in explanations of behaviour. I will also try to bring up to date the problem that Lashley regarded as a central issue in his experimental work, the question of how the brain operates successfully despite damage to its parts, as well as fragmentariness and variation of details of patterns on the retina.

I make no attempt at making complete presentations of empirical data. There are plenty of texts that tackle that task. Instead I concentrate on theories and explanations rather than experiments, and though I touch on some of the issues of learning and motivation, for the most part I shall use the issues of visual perception to carry the arguments forward.

Lashley very much gave the impression of having followed his own advice of the third quotation given above, and 'studied the brain itself'. As a result of this he was able to delineate at least some of the important conditions that must be fulfilled by theories of how the brain produces behaviour. Yet despite the fact that his advice is often good, I take exactly the opposite view to Lashley at this point, and will pursue more or less far-fetched analogies with machines of various kinds, particularly computers.

Though Lashley studied the brain and behaviour, and was an astute theoretician, I will argue that his principal difficulty was precisely that he was hampered by the lack of apt physical analogies for the processes he studied. His biological work hinted at the existence of principles of organization necessary for behaviour, and this work predated the understanding of any such principles embodied in physical systems. But these processes remained mysterious, because without making analogies with systems that we are already familiar with or can become familiar with, we find it difficult or impossible to grasp the unfamiliar brain. Analogies are theories, are explanations in familiar terms, are metaphors, are understandings. Without them studying the brain and behaviour may be tantalizing, but ultimately it is sterile. Somewhat more than twenty years after Lashley's death the 'similarities in such comparisons' with various kinds of machines may no longer be just the product of oversimplification, but may allow us to discern the nature of principles that make behaviour possible. Any understanding of the brain is a theory, is an analogy. Oversimplication has certainly occurred, and even to an absurd degree. No doubt it will continue. But not because analogies have been drawn from the latest fashion in physics. Rather it has taken place because the particular analogies or theories upon which brain researchers have drawn (apparently unconsciously at times) are too impoverished to give any insight into the workings of a complex brain. Lashley himself sought an apposite metaphor from the physical world, but the best he could come up with to give some idea of how it is the 'pattern and not the element that counts' was a system of diffraction patterns of waves on an inhomogeneous liquid. This is not just an arbitrary example of someone searching for the form of a theory by drawing on a metaphor from the furniture of our ordinary world. I will argue that this kind of physical analogy is typical, and that brain research has been continuously handicapped as much by the lack of sufficiently powerful metaphors or analogies as by any other factor. Now with the beginnings of understanding of how to create intelligent processes in computers we are armed with a set of analogies or metaphors altogether richer and more adequate for thinking about brain function than before.

Lashley was, of course, right to rail against oversimplification; and the oversimplification which he principally railed against was that of behaviour produced by reflex connections, conditioned or otherwise. We are now in a position to go further with the kind of theory that belatedly should replace the reflex, and as it happens the attempt to design aritficial intelligence in computers has helped to begin to see what form it should take, whether computers constitute the latest fashion in physics or not.

Chapters 2 and 3, amongst other things, involve an argument that in one important sense of the word 'understand' we only understand physiological mechanisms in so far as we have good psychological theories, i.e. theories of the logical structure of behaviour. The book thereafter concentrates upon matters in which we have some understanding of the necessary logical structure for particular types of behaviour or mental process, and I discuss how our psychological theories affect our interpretation of physiology.

A number of matters often considered to be part of physiological psychology, or brain research, or neurobiology, do not come within the scope of this account; I hope because they are either tangential to understanding behaviour and mental processes, or at best contribute to it only rather slightly. Thus the laborious pursuit of the conclusion that brain area A seems to have something to do with behaviour X or the research that allows us to admire the intricacy of some elaborate network in the brain without being able to say what it does or how it does it is not discussed to any large extent.

Two things which would seem appropriate in a book on physiological psychology would be to discuss first how known properties of neurones and neural nets might constrain, suggest and ultimately constitute explanations of how behaviour is produced, and second, how our understanding of mental processes and behaviour inform our understanding of their physiological embodiment. Though not dismissing the importance of this first concern, I concentrate largely on the second. These two seem to (or perhaps ought to) be principal concerns of physiological psychology.

Perhaps the central theme of the book is the exploration of how theory pervades scientific activity in brain research and, indeed, any activity. In brain research some kinds of experiment, e.g. recording electrical activity from a nerve cell, seem to lead to the conclusion that we can have direct contact with facts about the brain, without the impediment of theory or speculation which will necessarily distort or deceive: what we need to understand about the brain are plenty of these facts. I have tried to show within the context of brain research and experimental psychology that such a stance is shaky, if not misleading. To talk about such observations as facts is still to hold a theory, but a theory that is not expressed or even recognized as such is so much the worse for its non-recognition.

It may seem surprising but the implicit theory which still pervades most brain research and much psychology is the theory of reflexes, and this theory can be shown to be distinctly limited.

Reflex theory has had a good long run (more than 300 years) and we have by now understood quite a lot of its limitations. There are very many. Rather than pretending that the terms of this theory are fact, and at the same time being continually unable to come to grips with the more interesting aspects of the brain, what we need are new and better ways of thinking about the subject. Such ways are at last becoming available in a form that can be used.

2 *The brain as a physical system*

Lashley's prescription, as discussed briefly in chapter 1, was that in order to find out how the brain works we should study the brain itself. By this he presumably meant that in order to understand how the brain works to embody learning, perception, language, cognition and various other interesting, intelligent mental processes and behaviour, we should study the brain itself. Lashley made it clear in his work that he did not want to understand the brain as a factory for the manufacture of strange chemicals or a generator of electrical events. He, more clearly than most, saw one of the important tasks as explaining mind.

The basis on which such an attempt must rest for the scientist is the axiom that the brain is in some sense a physical system which supports or is somehow responsible for mind, and furthermore that we can deploy scientific methodology to attack it. In many ways the apparent truth of this axiom has grown steadily more complete (at least to the scientific mind) for the last 100 years. So much is this so that most scientists do not now doubt that the brain is the organ responsible for behaviour and mental processes. If it ceases physiological function, for instance, behaviour also stops.

In this context the acclaim given to many experiments relating the brain to some aspect of behaviour may seem a bit surprising: surprising because the main virtue of many of these experiments is that they seem to demonstrate mainly that some aspect of the physical brain is 'responsible for' or 'accompanies' some particular mental process or behaviour. Acclaim for many new discoveries seems, in other words, to be acclaim for yet a further demonstration that the brain is the seat of the mind. This conclusion is almost forced on one because of the real difficulty in seeing any other reason why a very large number of experiments on the brain should be regarded as 'interesting'.

I will illustrate this rather contentious argument by briefly describing a few physiological discoveries of different kinds that have captured attention to different degrees in the last twenty-five years.

1 *Self stimulation* Discovered by Olds and Milner in 1954; the phenomenon is that rats will learn to press a lever or perform some other action to deliver trains of electrical stimulation to particular regions of their brain, e.g. the lateral hypothalamus. This stimulation is evidently highly rewarding, rats generally prefer it to other forms of reward when offered the choice, and will continue to stimulate themselves in this way for many hours.

2 *Contingent negative variation* This is a slow negative shift in the baseline of an electroencephalographic recording (which is not seen using conventional EEG amplifiers in which baseline shifts are filtered out). It was discovered by Grey Walter *et al* (1964) and found to occur when an interval of several seconds occurred between a click and a series of flashes which the subject was required to stop by pressing a button. The negative wave seemed to correlate with the subject's expectancy, or anticipation of the flashes, but did not occur if the subject had decided not to press the button.

3 *Hand detectors* Gross *et al.* (1972) have discovered (in monkeys) neurones in the inferotemporal region that respond only when a primate hand is displayed in the animal's visual field.

4 *Dreaming* Jouvet (e.g. 1967) has claimed that the removal of parts of the hind-brain (the locus coeruleus) selectively abolishes the phase of sleep (the so-called phase of rapid eye movements) during which (in people) the majority of vivid dreams seem to occur.

5 *Stimulation of 'memories'* In the course of surgical procedures Penfield and Rasmussen (1950) applied electrical stimulation to the surface of the cortex in unanaesthetized patients. In a few locations, stimulation was said by the patient to evoke a vivid memory of a scene from his or her past.

6 *Physiological signs of meditation* Kasamatsu and Hirai (1966) have discovered that there are characteristic changes of electroencephalogram responses during deep meditational states in Zen Buddists.

Clearly one can not demonstrate that the impact of this or any other selection of discoveries is due to people being a bit surprised that the physical brain is intimately concerned with, and perhaps responsible for, behaviour or mental processes.

Arguable though it may seem, I find it difficult to escape the thought that this 'surprise' reaction is somehow due to the existence of things which we were perfectly convinced about in mental life, e.g. reward, expectancy, recognition of a hand, dreaming, vivid recall of a scene, or even meditation, being confirmed, and made somehow more real by demonstrating its accompaniment by some entirely physical process in an entirely physical organ.

It is slightly strange to suppose that quite real mental events should need to be reified by the discovery of some physiological correlate. It can be argued, or course, not perhaps that the discoveries themselves, but the subsequent use of the discovered physiological processes as tools in some further investigation of the mental processes, might have been, or might be productive of understandings. Yet these discoveries (striking as they apparently have been to many) do not often seem to have contributed much to our understanding of reward, dreaming, meditation, or whatever. Self-stimulation, for instance, discovered more than twenty years ago, has by now been followed by several thousand experiments on the technique. Tens of thousands of rats and other animals (and even a few people) have stimulated their own 'pleasure centres'. Though there has been this immense effort, experiments have been typically on the phenomenon of 'self-stimulation', and have not on the whole addressed issues such as the nature of reward, or the role of reward in learning or whatever, which one might think were important questions raised by the finding. Instead the basic question nowadays, to which twenty years of research has led, is whether self-stimulation is or is not like conventional rewards. As Tulving and Madigan (1972) have pointed out, yesterday's methods become today's objects of study. The answer in the case of self-stimulation seems to be that despite various oddities of behaviour associated with it, this artificial reward can be thought of as like a conventional one in many ways (see e.g. Trowell *et al*, 1969). Even when produced by electricity though, pleasure is not unalloyed. Some of the odd effects of self-stimulation could be due to the fact that a single stimulation is both pleasantly rewarding, and unpleasantly aversive (Kent and Grossman, 1970).

Part of the point seems to be that experiments which relate brain to behaviour seem to have some quality of showing that a very physical organ, the brain, which one can see and even stick one's thumb into, seems to be intimately connected with the much more mysterious and insubstantial matters of behaviour or mental processes. Yet the character of the demonstration is such that though they relate some part or activity of the brain to some aspect of behaviour, they do not seem of themselves to be able to illuminate the nature of the relation, or the structure of the mental process in question. They demonstrate the existence of a relationship more clearly than help us to understand it.

It may be that a continuous series of demonstrations of this kind is necessary. We do not know 'for certain' that mind is a purely physical matter. Scientists can certainly be encouraged by the various psycho-physiological relationships that have been demonstrated, since if psychology can be shown to depend on a physical brain then scientists are emboldened. Physical systems are precisely those which they have experience in investigating.

But besides the demonstrations, there are some further arguments as to why a physical basis for mental events seems plausible: arguments which, moreover, seem to open up better prospects for understanding mental processes. Two of the better ones are as follows:

The first, implicit in almost every testable hypothesis about the mechanism of the brain, was put particularly forcefully by Turing (1936). He defined a theoretical machine which occupied only discrete states. By being equipped with a potentially infinite input-output tape as a data and storage medium the number of states of the machine together with its stored data become infinite. One property of such machines is that they can be universal: considerations of speed apart, any one universal Turing machine can do what can be done by any other. Digital computers, the modern embodiment of the Turing machine are, therefore, called 'general purpose'. Any system that can be considered as existing in defined states, however numerous, can in principle be simulated by a computer. Amongst other things, this means that if we were able to define, that is to say, state exactly what the brain did in order to generate particular mental processes and behaviour, we could simulate these in a computer, and thus create mental processes in an entirely artificial device.

Some of the implications of this proposition for simulating mental processes were explored by Turing (1950). He proposed an imitation game, which incidentally was one of the first contributions to the field of artificial intelligence. In the game a human player sits at a teletypewriter, and via this device he or she interrogates two respondents, another person and a digital computer. The player's task is to say which is which. There is now no serious doubt that at some time in the future it will become possible to play Turing's imitation game, and that it will prove to be difficult over limited periods at least, and perhaps within limited domains of discourse, to tell the difference between a human and a suitably programmed computer.

Objections have been made to the programs which have so far been written and which do already play a version of Turing's game; (e.g. Weizenbaum, 1965) that they perform only by a series of tricks which do not represent the way human beings think.

Consider for instance the following exchanges related by Bobrow (1970). One Saturday morning a vice president of a company in charge of selling computer services arrived at a computing laboratory at MIT hoping to demonstrate the computing system to a potential customer. He found a note on the teletypewriter which read 'TYPE ALL MESSAGES INTO THIS TELETYPE, AND END THEM WITH A FULL STOP.' This note had been left by one of the programmers who had been using a version of Weizenbaum's program. The program was in fact designed to produce responses that a non-directive psychotherapist might make to a client. The vice-president (VP) however thought that the note indicated that the teletype was connected to Bobrow's home, since Bobrow often used the computer from a terminal at his home during the night. Therefore, the VP started, as he thought, talking to Bobrow, though he was actually connected to Weizenbaum's computer program, and the following conversation ensued.

VP:	DO YOU THINK THAT I CAN USE THE COMPUTER THIS MORNING?
Teletype response:	WHY DO YOU ASK?
VP:	I MIGHT BE ABLE TO MAKE SOME ADDITIONAL TELECOMP SALES.
Teletype response:	WHY AREN'T YOU SURE?
VP:	MY PROSPECTIVE CUSTOMERS HAVE NEVER SEEN A DEMONSTRATION OF THE SYSTEM.

Teletype response: DOES THIS MEAN VERY MUCH TO YOU?
VP: OF COURSE IT DOES.
Teletype response: YOU SEEM VERY POSITIVE ABOUT THAT.
VP: THIS IS RIDICULOUS.
Teletype response: WHAT DO YOU MEAN THIS IS RIDICULOUS?
VP: IS THERE ANY REASON WHY I CAN'T USE THE COMPUTER NOW?
Teletype response: TELL ME MORE ABOUT YOUR PROSPECTIVE CUSTOMERS.
VP: PLEASE DIAL ME UP ON 491-1850.

After this last remark, the VP did not obey the instruction to terminate each message with a full stop, and the computer therefore did not respond. This so infuriated the poor VP that he phoned up Bobrow, waking him from a deep sleep and said:

VP: Why are you being so snotty to me?
Bobrow: What do you mean why am I being snotty to you?

The VP angrily read back the conversation to Bobrow, who collapsed with laughter, and apparently it took him some time to explain to the VP that he had been talking to the computer.

Weizenbaum's program works by picking up certain key words in the human input messages and using these to respond either with a transformed version of the immediately preceding or some earlier input, often in a question form (e.g. WHAT DO YOU MEAN THIS IS RIDICULOUS?), or responding with some question of a more general kind. It reminds one of the well known joke 'Why do you always answer a question with a question?' 'So why shouldn't I answer and question with a question?' The cirticism that it works by tricks and evasions is thus to some extent just, but it misses a number of important points.

A significant point in this context is that to the extent that the simulation is successful the states of a system capable of generating that kind of behaviour must have been defined, and thus made capable of being simulated by a Turing machine. In so far as the computer can simulate acceptably human behaviour, it becomes less pressing to suppose that we need to postulate some non-physical basis for producing that kind of behaviour. Moreover, Weizenbaum's program does contain certain kinds of knowledge about conversations which make it possible for the conversations to be held e.g. that the conversants take turns, and may refer to what has gone before. It seems that people, too, must use this same kind of knowledge when they converse. Thus such programs, although incomplete, do demonstrate principles that make certain mental processes possible.

A different argument for a physical basis of mind due to Craik (1943) implied that a brain could work perfectly well if it were to obey only physical principles. He stated that for the brain to perform its known functions it must represent in symbolic form the causal and other relationships of the environment. The brain amongst other things must be a model of the physical world. Such a working model could predict the events that are likely to occur in the world. Often only by prediction of what will occur can appropriate behaviour be generated. Thus according to Craik, thought parallels reality through symbolism. Neural symbolic processes reflect laws such as those of causality obtaining in the environment. Applying Turing's principles again, since defined physical processes can represent each other, in order to simulate the physical world, the brain could probably do no better than to use physical principles of operation to do so.

McCulloch and Pitts (1943) put a similar proposition in their paper published in the same year as Craik's monograph. They expressed these points in a more exact fashion: symbolic descriptions of sequences of events may be embodied in finite nets of formal neurons. McCulloch and Pitts went further than this, however, and outlined a proof of the relation of neural nets to Turing's abstract computers. Neural nets (or formal neurones) plus receptors and effectors are equivalent to Turing-machines.

If the brain did not simulate, and indeed embody in symbolic form, the relationships of the real world (by computing, for instance, the likelihood of external events) animals would be unlikely to achieve their biological goals. The manner in which we perform even mundane acts such as getting out of a chair, walking, running to catch a bus and so on, indicates that our brains contain a representation of the spatio-temporal relationships of the world in which we live.

Without such representations, we should have to try out a large number of alternative haphazard acts each time an undetermined situation was reached because we would not know what led to what. A trial-and-error search for adaptive behaviour may well have taken place in natural selection. But this process has now resulted in a brain that contains rather specific facilities for constructing more or less adequate representations of the external world. These mechanisms are capable of assimilating selected information, for instance about temporal and spatial relationships between events, so that further trial and error search by the individual is minimized.

One may, with Chomsky (e.g. Chomsky and Hampshire, 1968) regard the whole issue of whether there is a physical basis for mental activity as rather an empty one. Chomsky argues that 'historically the term "physical" has been extended step by step to cover anything we understand'. However, we do not know whether currently understood physical and physiological processes are capable of being extended to explain all mental activity, and this is an empirical question (Sutherland, 1970). Despite Chomsky's dismissal of the issue, it is, nevertheless, important for scientists (including Chomsky) to have a belief that the brain is in some sense a physical, or at least an understandable, system. Otherwise the methodology of science would not be equal to dealing with it and the whole exercise would be something of a waste of time. What we can say is that already brain research and artificial intelligence have indicated that some areas of behaviour can in principle be understood along physical lines, and no convincing *a priori* arguments have been advanced which indicate that this understanding cannot continue.

It is certainly true that in detail present computers and people differ in many respects. With very few exceptions, computers have so far been programmed only to perform a limited range of very specific tasks, whereas people are able to attack a wide variety of different problems by seeing the important elements, relationships and causal chains that are involved. The parallel processing of signals by the human visual system is completely unmatched by any computer system. A list of 'differences' could be extended indefinitely. Nevertheless the computer is the only 'physical' system that now exists in which any intellectual tasks at all can be artificially created, and programs which perform such tasks display capacities hitherto thought to be solely human. Computers and brains are at least comparable in that they are both complex knowledge using devices.

Computer programs have already been constructed to have quite complex models or representations of at least limited environments. One problem which I shall take up further is that these programs function in such a fashion as to make at least some kinds of experimental analysis of their operation into 'elementary' functional units very difficult.

Discussion about the relation of brains to computers has most often revolved around the problem of whether, even at their most intelligent, machines could ever really think. At a recent conference the question as to whether a computer might one day be qualified to enter the Kingdom of Heaven was even put. Fascinating though discussions of the status of a computer able to play Turing's game impeccably might by, they miss the point. The problem is not about the nature of the computer. This we know. It is a discrete state machine, obeying moderately well understood laws of physics. What we do not know is the nature of the brain.

It seems likely that by continuing to experiment with knowledge using representational processes in computers, we may be able to discern common principles between effective programs and mental processes. In so doing, we use whatever commonality there is between computers and brains to give ourselves better metaphors, better ways of thinking about the mind, than the even less adequate physical metaphors such as 'ripples on the surface of a liquid'. Nobody would suppose that a liquid could think. At least there is some question as to whether computers can.

3 *Techniques of brain research and the questions they answer*

If we are taking a scientific route to understanding the mind, it follows that we are prepared to see the task perhaps as ridiculously difficult, but essentially as a 'physical' problem in the sense I have discussed. Those scientists attempting to find out how the brain works therefore have a task which though daunting could in principle be soluble. However, it is instructive to wonder whether techniques currently used to attack the brain would be equal to investigating a much simpler system, which handles symbolic information, i.e. a digital computer. Finding out how the computer works (a different kind of Turing game) might well give us some insight into the nature of the observations that can be made in brain research. It tells us what kind of information could be obtained from the exercise of the different available techniques. It helps, in short, to understand some of the strengths and weaknesses of the various methods used in brain research. The argument depends not on any detailed similarity between computer and brain but merely upon the fact that both are devices which manipulate symbolic knowledge and in that sense have properties in common.

A NEW COMPUTER GAME

The game is played somewhat as follows. Let us suppose that we are given an unlimited number of similar large computers, typically consisting of central processors and store, input and output machinery including for example a visual display, and an extensive library of programs (the software). Suppose that we are allowed to use only the techniques now available to biologists and psychologists who work on the brain to investigate this species of computer. How should we proceed in order to discover exactly how it works, given only that we know it to be a symbol manipulating system? We should not, of course, be allowed to consult the designers or the software writers.

First here is a summary of some of the techniques used to investigate the brain. We can then see how these might be applied to a computer.

1 Anatomy. The description of the structure of the brain and its parts, including the presentation of photographs and diagrams of its elements and their interconnections: methods for determining the connectivity of various widely spaced elements are included.

2 Biophysics and biochemistry. The study of subcellular structures and mechanisms, such as the neuronal membrane.

3 Neurophysiology. The investigation by means of stimulation and electrical recording, and by means of selective lesions, of the (mainly) local activity of parts of the brain, with emphasis on the activity of what seems to be the simplest functional element, the neurone: the investigation of the responses of neurones and neuronal aggregates to stimuli.

4 Psychology. The study of input-output relationships of basically intact animals, including the study of human mental processes and behaviour.

5 Physiological psychology. The study of the behaviour not of intact animals, but of those which have been physiologically prepared by electrical biochemical or surgical techniques.

6 Ethology. The study of animals' behaviour in their natural environment and their behavioural adaptation to that environment.

7 Theoretical studies. The study of mathematical, logical and computer models of various physiological and psychological phenomena for the purpose of quantifying, predicting and explaining the activity and functioning of the brain.

What would be our present state of knowledge about the computer if techniques of the kind listed above had been applied to computers over a period comparable to that during which brain research has been taking place?

Anatomy

Conventional anatomical techniques would certainly have furnished descriptions of a number of types of computer-component, recognizable on the basis of shape, size and colour. Their interconnectors – thin, flat, bright metal strips over short ranges, brightly coloured plastic-coated wires over longer ranges would also be clear. Some important features of circuit organization might have been discovered, such as the existence of tracts (bundles of wires) and nuclei (conglomerations of components). On the other hand, anatomists might well have paid altogether too much attention to such a prominent object as the circuit-board which can easily be removed and replaced, but which is not necessarily of profound physiological significance but indicates rather that it is convenient to place in close proximity on the same small board, circuits which are to be interconnected. The circuit-board as a unit of anatomical organization might have misled anatomists for some time into neglecting very much more functionally significant structures, such as the bi-stable circuit (a switch capable of existing electrically in two defined states) which underlies the binary logic of the computer. Especially with integrated circuits it might have proved extremely difficult anatomically to recognize the bi-stable as a fundamental unit, though with the help of biophysics this could be done. The difference between an easily recognizable anatomical structure of no great significance, and one with clearer functional significance recalls the difference between the classical anatomical description of the cortex as being layered (e.g. Sholl, 1956) and its apparent functional organization into columns (Hubel and Wiesel, 1962).

It can be assumed, therefore, that comparative anatomical studies of the structure of today's computers, together with studies of their precursors would have resulted in a reasonably comprehensive description of their structural organization, but without necessarily any deep insight into their functional organization.

A further type of collaboration between anatomy and biophysics might be in the electron-microscopy of circuit elements, which may have been correlated with the biophysical properties of the components. Thus the role of the very thin dielectric layer of a capacitor in storing charge may well have been understood.

Biophysics

It is very probable that computer biophysicists would have made significant discoveries concerning the structure and functions of some basic computer circuit elements. The resistor, the capacitor, the ferrite ring and so forth would have had their properties rather fully investigated, and the electrical pulses by means of which information is apparently transmitted between the various parts of the computer would also have been described in great detail. The most exciting and important discoveries would no doubt have concerned small bi-stable circuits which would have been found to obey an all-or-none law. As a function of the voltage at the input terminal, the output voltage would be seen to exist at only two fundamental levels. There might also be a good deal of enthusiasm for the hypotheses that two main types of transistor were to be found. The operation of one type might be explained by supposing that it conducts by means of the transfer of positive charges while the other would be thought to transfer negative charges.

While nobody would deny that work on computer biophysics was of great elegance and precision, and that several of the major discoveries would rightly deserve the highest praise, opinion as to the importance of this type of enquiry for any final understanding of computers would be divided. Some would believe that only by understanding the electronic mechanisms in detail could any satisfactory understanding of the computer as a whole be reached, while others would doubt whether study of mechanisms at this atomic level would reveal any fundamental principles of the operation of the computer as a system.

Neurophysiology

The computer neurophysiologist, working at a rather more molar level might well have been proceeding somewhat as follows. He might have opened up the cabinet of his computer with a can opener, mounted a long probe onto a lowering device situated over the opening, and, perhaps referring to a map of the inner structure (provided by a computer-anatomist), lowered the probe gently into the innards. The probe would be fairly tough and rigid, insulated except for the tip which might be about the size of a pin-point. Recording the voltage between this tip and (say) the outer surface of the cabinet, the neurophysiologist would advance the probe until he saw on his oscilloscope the signs of some well-defined electrical activity, such as pulses. He might then stimulate the computer by means of the teletype, and record the resulting pulse patterns seen on the oscilloscope. He might calculate (with another computer?) various statistics associated with the pulse patterns; interval histograms, post-stimulus time histograms, and if he had two or more probes, cross-correlograms. Computer neurophysiology would in fact have produced a huge amount of data on the firing patterns of various circuit elements and configurations: the input-output behaviour of circuit-boards might have been established, and the average responses of tracts and nuclei would have been described.

Solid achievements of the computer neurophysiologists might be the recognition of something of the informational significance of bi-stable circuits. When these alter from state to state rapidly, they are responding to some input, so that it would be possible to tell that particular bi-stables responded to particular patterns of input. Despite the field's prestige, however, there would be very considerable difficulties of interpreting data.

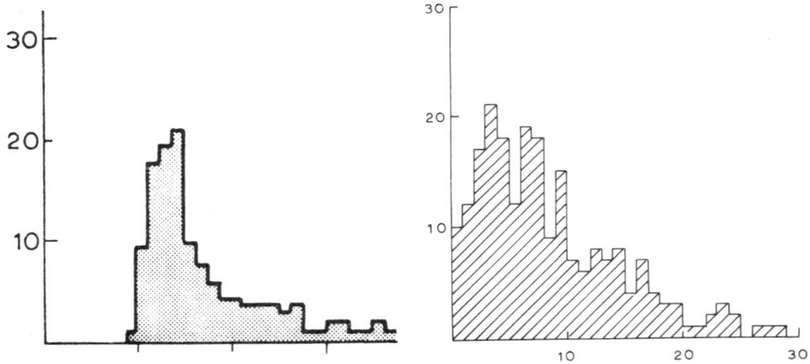

Figure 3.1 Interval histograms: (a) from a neurone (Burns, 1968) and (b) of the letter 'e' in a passage of prose. Whereas the neurone has a refractory period the letter 'e' does not, otherwise the histograms are not dissimilar.

Interval histograms from single bi-stable units might look rather like the ones produced from neurones (fig. 3.1a), or even like the one shown in fig. 3.1b. The histogram in fig. 3.1b was computed (in effect) by monitoring the letter 'e' of a computer teletypewriter, and plotting the frequency of occurrence of that letter against the intervals between its occurrence when the message was a passage from *Alice's Adventures in Wonderland*. It is evident that although the unit is clearly selective for a particular pattern of input, no amount of sophisticated analysis of this firing pattern would give any information about the actual message being transmitted. Monitoring the activity of many of the other types of single unit would be similarly difficult to interpret since knowing the distribution of events in a single bi-stable of a computer is going to be of no help in understanding what role that unit has in the mechanism. Particularly in many redundant, and error-correcting codes, information is carried in the relationships between the individual elements not in any individual elements.

Another reason for supposing that studies of individual components might not have turned out to be as productive of important knowledge about computers as one might think is that, under the circumstances in which most recordings would have been made, only a small population of unrepresentative components might have been studied. In order to carry out microelectrode experiments the computer physiologist would have found how to make the computer run in such a way that he could record something reasonably often. In order to obtain exact and reproducible results he would have tended to put the computer into operating modes that produced continuous activity for fairly long periods. No doubt, techniques for doing this would have been discovered, just as animal neurophysiologists have found that certain anaesthetics are useful for this purpose. To maintain suitable continuous activity in the computer one could run a program consisting of a loop. But the repetition, though conforming to scientific standards of reproducibility, can only be seen as a not particularly representative mode of the computer's behaviour. Indeed, if there is no exit from the loop towards an output of information, then this activity might well be termed 'unphysiological' or even 'pathological'. The point of these remarks is that there are limits to the circumstances in which microelectrode recordings will yield useful knowledge. Some specification of the connections of the unit under study is required, and even more important, some insight into the significance (for the unit) of the signals which are being transmitted. Such requirements are more likely to be met near that part of the machine which receives inputs than anywhere else. It is therefore to be expected that a great deal of information concerning computer peripherals would have accumulated as a result of such studies, including perhaps some classification of the set of adequate stimuli: those stimuli that serve to elicit well-defined but not necessarily well understood changes of state in the computer. But real insights into how components were involved in signalling or symbol manipulation processes might easily not have been achieved.

Psychology

On the assumption that the computer had a full load of resident programs, psychologists would have carried out an investigation of the behaviour of the computer, i.e. they would have searched for those inputs that elicit responses from the computer. The complete set of such inputs might not have been discovered but it can be assumed that some sort of subset would have been found. Thus the input 'PRINT' 3;, coded and punched onto card or paper-tape, might have been discovered to cause the on-line teletypewriter to write 3. The further discovery that inputs of the kind 'PRINT' 3 + 2; caused the teletypewriter to write 5 would have led to the discovery that the computer could perform addition. In this way one primary objective of the psychological experiments would have been approached, namely the operational definition of the abilities of the computer; a specification of its behaviour together with antecedent conditions. Finally, some account of the user-language of the computer might have been painstakingly assembled, following a great many linguistic manipulations.

While descriptions of input-output relations were being compiled some psychologists would also be performing experiments to elucidate lower level software, determining the logical organization of the machine. Probably only rather limited progress would have been made in this direction, with the unfortunate consequence that the computer neurophysiologists would be very much in the dark, both as to the types of operations that assemblies of basic units might perform, and as to the meaning for the machine of most types of input signals.

The difficulties with many of the hypotheses entertained by computer psychologists might be that though often ingenious, after a good deal of very careful experimentation they would turn out to be wrong. One psychological theory, clearly plausible and held for some time, might be that division was performed by the computer by means of successive subtractions. This hypothesis would predict that for any dividend the time taken to perform a division would be proportional to the size of the divisor. Because of the relative crudity of early psychological measurement techniques this hypothesis might be difficult to test. Indications that division always took longer than subtraction would be regarded as encouraging, but more exact measurements would show that the time taken was more nearly constant than proportional to the size of the divisor. Notwithstanding these difficulties, psychologists might continue to invent ways in which the computer might translate the higher level languages into structures of lower level machine commands. At very least, a number of logical operations that might have been used by the computer would have been shown by psychological experiments not to be used.

Physiological Psychology

The aim of computer physiological psychology would be to identify and explain the mechanisms of systems in terms somewhere between the atomic and the molar. One of the first tasks might be conceived as collaboration with anatomists to identify which parts of the computer are responsible for particular behavioural functions. The techniques used might involve some kind of experimental manipulation of the inside of the computer combined with observation of the output of the normal peripheral devices. Computer lesion techniques for instance would have been much used in the hope of finding out whether particular parts of the machine were involved in particular types of behaviour. These would include cutting cable tracts, removing circuit boards, and for larger scale operations removing substantial quantities of the computer with a shovel. For the finer work deep inside the computer, probes of much the same kind as those used by the computer neurophysiologist would be placed accurately into some part of the machine. Instead of a recording tip these probes could carry a small explosive charge, about the size of a fire-cracker, to be detonated remotely. This tiny bomb would produce localized destruction in regions difficult to reach by other methods. These lesion techniques might be supplemented by means whereby large voltages can be applied to different parts of the machine (electrical stimulation) and by 'pharmacological' manipulations such as changing the power supply voltages. Many of these operations would have dramatic effects on the behaviour of the machine.

The outcome of these experiments would, however, be difficult to interpret. It might be believed that some areas of the computer are more important for certain functions than others. Some types of storage or symbol manipulation, for instance, might have been 'localized', whereas there would be some areas where any kind of damage seems to produce failure of the machine to perform any behaviour whatever.

Ethology

The fact that the computers in question simply arrived mysteriously in brain research laboratories would unfortunately deprive investigators of one important kind of information about them, the nature of their behaviour in the environment for which they were designed. Despite the experimental methodology which has enabled empirical determination of the abilities of organisms, knowing what they typically do, what tasks they typically have to undertake and what problems of interactions with the environment they solve, is information of a fundamental kind. Computers are not yet robots, and the spontaneous interactions with the world of the specimens provided so far would be very limited.

Theoretical Studies

It is perhaps easier to predict what theories might have developed concerning computer organization and function, for we might have theories of automata, information and control already to draw upon. Given, however, that theorists were not party to the design of our computers, we might not expect much of a theory concerning list processing operations, nor very much detailed insight into the basic details of computer organization, save perhaps for a general recognition of the analogies between computers and desk calculating machines. The relation between hardware and software might be ill-understood. There might, however, be a considerable logical and statistical theory of the organization and activity of computer components and circuits, and the properties of networks of computer-like components might be well understood mathematically through analogue simulation. More recently use of these simulated components might have developed a branch of enquiry known as artificial computation, in which an attempt was made to reproduce some of the more complicated computer-like functions using man-made devices.

STRUCTURE AND EXPLANATION

This rather light-hearted account of a few methods used in brain research and the way in which they might be transposed if applied to certain computers that might have appeared in brain research laboratories throughout the world, or if one imagined a race of intelligent machines investigating themselves, does not exhaust the available techniques. Biochemical methods, for instance, are very prominent in brain research at present. As well as being applied to problems where subcellular events are the main ones of interest, they are also used in physiological psychology where behavioural responses to biochemical manipulations are at issue.

This rather fanciful allegory is not meant to imply that present-day computers are like brains in any detail. In fact, they are unlike brains in many ways. For instance, the all-or-nothing activity of neurones, which has been thought to be similar to the digital binary logic of computers is clearly no such thing; the main information we have indicates a role of nerve impulse traffic in some form of pulse-interval modulation coding, an analogue representation. Also the completely sequential operation of present-day computers is quite unlike much of the activity of brains. These and other differences do not, however, prevent the putting of general propositions about how one might approach any complex device that processes symbolic information. The analogy is meant to illustrate shortcomings of some of the methods used in brain research and to suggest what kind of information is most fruitfully sought by using different methods: what, in other words, are the observables? It rests not on detailed similarities between computers and brains, but on some general properties of devices that can manipulate symbols and generate behaviour.

It seems straightforward to suppose that the first preliminary steps towards an understanding of how computers and brains work involve some knowledge of their composition and behaviour; structure and function. In this respect anatomy and psychology are primary. The basically anatomical notion that by opening a mechanism up and inspecting its innards we shall be able to see how it works is a compelling one. When we know the properties of parts and can see the ways in which parts interact, perhaps also giving the works a push here or a prod there, then we can sometimes get a good idea about the mechanism.

But for many kinds of interaction direct vision is impossible, so that for instance the strategy of opening it up and peering at it is not much good for finding out how a radio works. One might argue that we substitute for vision the measurement of voltages at various points. But this gives just pin-point estimates of activity at very local spots. Our considerable abilities of perceiving and understanding Gestalt patterns, which can be brought to bear on purely mechanical devices such as complicated pieces of clockwork, are lost. We have to substitute the more difficult procedures of logical analysis, complete with externalized aids such as mathematics, and we have painstakingly and slowly to construct new mental schemata for understanding electronic components such as capacitors and transistors, and yet other ones for circuits such as oscillators and amplifiers. Partly, of course, the purpose of neurophysiology and physiological psychology is to provide an understanding of the properties of neurones, and the properties of small groups of them in functionally specific arrangements. But it seems unlikely that this will be achieved without some specification of what the functions in question might be.

Lashley (1957) quotes an anecdote of his youth: when working as a research assistant he was sorting out some Golgi slides of the frog's brain and it occurred to him that he should 'work out all the connections among the cells so that we might know how the frog works'. But even if we had the technical ability to achieve a complete map of all the interconnections of neurones in the brain, we would not have solved the problem. Just as someone lacking the cognitive schemata for understanding a circuit diagram of some piece of electronic apparatus would make nothing of it, we would make nothing of such a neural wiring diagram, because we do not have the appropriate functional understandings.

The mistake we make in supposing that we can see how anything works by opening it up and looking at it is that this technique only works for purely mechanical devices. There it works partly because we have highly sophisticated schemata for mechanical interactions involving pushes and pulls, action and movement, levers and cogs. Some of these schemata, or theories, may be innate or learned very early by picking things up and moving about, and have to do with living in a world where many actions involve mechanisms. The success of looking to see how a mechanism works is also due to the fact that an operation, e.g. the pressure on a lever, produces a movement, a perceivable event. Part of the trouble with understanding for instance electronic processes is that we have no naive schemata for them, nor are causes followed by 'directly' perceivable events. There is before we have learned electronics nothing to connect our readings of instruments to actions or layout. In the brain, acquiring these functional schemata or theories as to how neural processes might produce behaviour is, of course, part of what the problem is all about.

A rather different problem which also bedevils our attempts at explanation of brain mechanisms is that of the different levels of explanation.

The relationship between these different levels of explanation has been illustrated in a simple way by Gregory (1961), see fig. 3.2. The block diagram approach at the most molar level

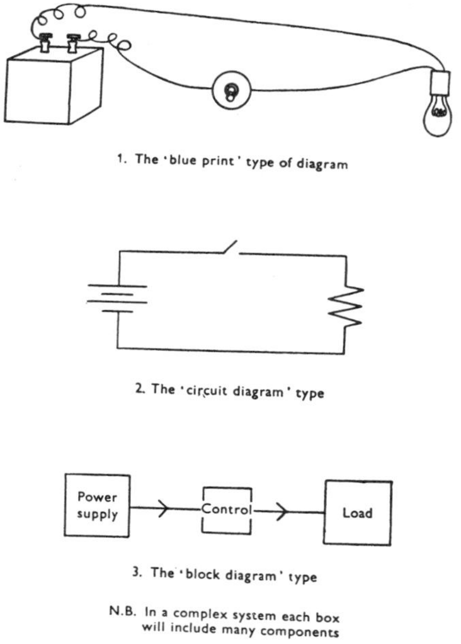

1. The 'blue print' type of diagram
2. The 'circuit diagram' type
Power supply
Control
Load
3. The 'block diagram' type
N.B. In a complex system each box will include many components

Figure 3.2 Different levels of description and explanation for an electric lighting system (from Gregory, 1961).

corresponds to one level of psychological enquiry, and is equivalent in the computer analogy to information flow diagrams and software generally. In the computer there are layers of progressively more atomic descriptions, high-level user languages, assembly language, machine code, logic diagrams and at the lowest level the circuit diagrams and the operational characteristics of circuit elements. In Gregory's example the lowest levels correspond to the circuit or wiring diagram. With complicated organizations a very large number of interrelated levels of description is absolutely necessary for any satisfactory understanding.

Descriptions somewhere between the most molar and the atomic represented by neurophysiology and physiological psychology can only be successful if related to descriptions above and below them in the hierarchy. One can occasionally hear from psychologists a despairing conclusion that this or that problem will have to await investigation by physiologists. Usually just the opposite is true. Physiologists are often (if not usually) unable to interpret their data without insights into the behavioural function of the mechanisms they are studying. In the aspect of the central nervous system investigated with the greatest success by physiologists, namely sensory systems, understanding of physiological phenomena has been due to more than a century's work in visual and auditory psychology and psychophysics, together with a good deal of insight about the functions of the systems derived from our own experiences of using vision and hearing. In the elucidation of many of the fundamental concepts in modern neurophysiology (synapses, receptive fields, adequate stimuli, etc), Sherrington's 'psychological' (1906) experiments and explanations preceded investigation at the level of individual neurones.

This hierarchical arrangement of levels of understanding seems essential for our comprehension of the brain. Each level of description expresses the logical organization of the system in terms of how components with defined properties interact at that level, and each level is reducible to another level of logical description at which it is explained why components at the higher level have the input-output relations they do. This continues down to the 'circuit diagram' level in which circuit elements are in fact lower-level blocks or boxes defined entirely by their properties, i.e. by an operational definition of their input-output relation. Though in electronics the symbol:

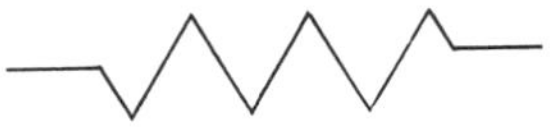

in a circuit diagram might suggest a small cylindrical object with wires protruding from it (a resistor), strictly speaking it does not signify anything tangible at all. Merely it states that the current through that part of the circuit is directly proportional to the voltage across it. Indeed, any diagram that can be made of the system except for an anatomical one, e.g. a blueprint, is necessarily a logical or conceptual diagram or model. In a complicated system understanding can only be achieved when there is a hierarchy of conceptual diagrams. And blocks at any given level are reducible to combinations of lower level blocks.

Despite this possibility of successive reduction to lower levels of explanation, the idea that because in the end all our explanations of the brain might be reducible to biophysical and biochemical events, we would therefore deduce from biophysical understandings how the brain works is quite false. If the properties of the brain depend on the organizational arrangement of components at lower levels, then it is not so much the properties of the parts themselves, but the various arrangements of parts which are important. The Gestalt adage that the whole is more than the sum of its parts is precisely true in that arrangements of interacting parts have properties which the parts themselves do not have, and which are not implicit in the nature of the parts, but arise out of their interactions. Examples of this are numerous, for instance the properties of a feedback circuit are not deducible just from the components that compose it (see chapter 5 for further discussion). Or as Weiss (1967) has pointed out, some rather exotic patterns of very similar form occur in nature, e.g. the tree-like branching patterns which appear in a neurone, a river, cracks in ice, blood vessels, and indeed trees, result not just from the properties of the components or physical materials of these phenomena, but from rather similar types of interactions between components: components in the various cases being quite dissimilar.

It is precisely the notion of emergent properties derived from the arrangement and organization of parts that makes necessary (for our understanding) the description of complex systems at a number of conceptual levels. If all the properties of a system were deducible from the properties of its parts alone, then all we would need to understand would be the fundamental particles of physics — and the whole universe and its workings would be understood.

Thus although a system with higher level properties is constructed of a particular set of physical parts, and although the properties of each part might be explicable in terms of properties of the arrangement of its constituents, this is not the same as saying that higher level properties can be deduced from or subsumed under properties of constituents alone. Otherwise we might deduce (say) the human behaviour of buying fish and chips from the properties of protons and electrons, or be able to describe entirely in the language of particle physics, how it is possible to understand this sentence.

To say that levels of explanation are necessary for our understanding is all very well, but there are immense difficulties in grappling with the complexity that is implied by multi-level organizations, particularly when the levels do not necessarily exist in the brain itself, but are defined by our attempts to organize the brain in such a way that we can understand it.

What this means for experimentation is that we must continually beware of confusions among the levels of explanation at which we work. For instance, there is a sense in which biophysicists have an advantageous position in operating principally within only one level of explanation, and with a good armoury of conceptual schemata supplied from well understood mechanisms of physics and chemistry. A further advantage is that biophysicists can utilize electrical pulses to activate a neurone from which they are recording. This is entirely appropriate because such pulses imitate the electrical changes that are the unit's normal input, and, therefore, provide a means of generating messages exactly similar to those which the unit normally responds to. This situation then is similar to that of psychology where input to, and output from, the experimental preparation is via the normal channels of perception and behaviour. However, for experiments between the levels of biophysics and psychology, that is for any large or ill-defined group of neurones, artificially generated electrical pulses do not provide a stimulus of which the meaning is known. Indeed, as far as the neural network is concerned the stimulus may be quite meaningless. Nor when recording the response of neurones to natural events is it evident merely from looking at the output of a cell what transformations of the messages have taken place. The temptation is to suppose that because electrical stimulation or a natural event causes repeatable and measurable changes in a neurophysiological network, that the change will be comprehensible. If the stimulation is at one conceptual level, and the recording at another, then the explanation of the experiment needs to cross the conceptual levels, and that is precisely what our present theories are too undeveloped to do. We may observe something measurable and repeatable, but we cannot so directly see its significance.

The wide range of levels of explanation implies that for the construction of theory, while we continually attempt to explain something at any given level in terms of the properties and interactions of components at a lower level, at least three things must be available. First, a good understanding of what the components and their properties at the lower level are; secondly, some good, functional description of what behaviour or properties are being produced, and thirdly, a set of conceptions about how the lower level components can be put together to produce the emergent properties or behaviour at the higher level.

It is clear that since an emergent property is not deducible from the properties of the components themselves our theories about them must come from somewhere else. Typically they come from inventions of one sort or another, often from outside the immediate biological situation. Thus our understanding of the spread of post-synaptic potentials along a dendrite comes from an engineering understanding of distributed capacitive and resistive properties of a cable. Biophysics is quite successful precisely because we have got both a good grasp of the properties of components (ions, solutions, membranes, and so on) and a set of ways of thinking about the interactions of such components provided by electronic engineering, chemistry and physics.

Biophysics, moreover, clearly supplies an understanding of the properties of components to the next level, neurophysiology. But without a set of concepts or ways of thinking about the interactions of elements at this next level, i.e. neurones, to draw upon, the process of inventing neurophysiological theories is slow. Invention seems to be the right word because a mechanism with an emergent property, not being simply deducible from its parts, must be invented. The main problem then seems to be whether we have a rich and fertile store of analogies, metaphors and models to draw on in order to help the process of inventing theories of interactions of components. Unfortunately, the more complex the behaviour and interactions we have to explain, and the further they are from our familiar world of actions and causes among solid objects disposed in space, the more inadequate is our ready-made set of conceptions about how such behaviour can be produced, the more we need new conceptual schemata, and ideas that we can import from elsewhere.

In brain research we must keep each of our explanatory levels supplied from below with a specification of functional components, their properties, and possibilities for interaction with each other. From above we must keep it supplied with descriptions of behaviour to be achieved. Perhaps, most important, we need a repertoire of ways of thinking about how complex and meaningful symbolic operations can be achieved.

EXPERIMENTAL BRAIN LESIONS AND STIMULATION

With physiological psychology the situation is particularly difficult. Although description at this level is constrained both by what is psychologically known and what is neurophysiologically possible, it is at this level that the complicated relationship between brain software and brain hardware is investigated and the logic underlying some of the attempts is often not clear. For instance, with the two favourite techniques of physiological psychology, lesions and stimulation, conclusions are drawn with various degrees of justification. First, it is often said that any behaviour not affected by stimulation or by lesions at a locus in the brain does not necessarily involve the circuits at that locus. Secondly, it is said that any behaviour affected by the lesion or the stimulation must normally require participation of that particular part of the brain. The second point needs qualification since a relatively unimportant part of the normal mechanisms might have an overwhelming pathological effect. A third conclusion is that a combination of stimulations and lesions will lead to the specification of areas in the brain that are both necessary and sufficient for any given category of behaviour. A fourth claim is that deviations from normal patterns of behaviour can provide information about the mechanisms underlying normal brain mechanisms.

Gregory (1961) has put a number of arguments against the

use of the lesion technique, specifically against the proposition that behaviour of a lesioned system helps us to understand the mechanisms producing normal behaviour. In a system where there is a high degree of interaction between the units or component parts as in the brain, there need be no simple relationship between the bizarre behaviour generated by an essentially pathological specimen with a lesion, and the functional organizations that generate normal behaviour. Often, explanations derived from lesion experiments are not explanations at all, but merely lightly disguised and not necessarily insightful descriptions of the behaviour produced under the influence of the lesion. Gregory illustrates this by saying that if a condenser (capacitor) fails within a radio set, causing the set to emit a piercing howl, we should surely not wish to argue that 'the normal function of the condenser is to inhibit howling'. Despite this it is easy to find reports of experiments that explain an animal's failure to stop responding to a negative stimulus in a discrimination task in terms of the destruction of a proposed inhibitory system.

The difficulty is that the argument for the strategy of removing things to see what happens is at first sight quite a plausible one. It seems first to have been put by Hughlings-Jackson (see collected works, 1958) and has been succinctly restated more recently by Teitelbaum (1967) as follows: 'The bizarre symptoms we see after brain damage always help us to understand normal behaviour.' Not only do lesions split behaviour into simpler components, runs the argument, but the abnormal reveals the normal. Bizarre behaviour following brain lesions is nothing more than an exaggeration of aspects of normal behaviour; the lesion provides us with a sort of behavioural magnifying glass.

There certainly seems to be an air of logic in the supposition that the components which produce the pathological behaviour must be those which are present normally but freed from the controlling influence of damaged parts, or as Hughlings-Jackson states 'pathological symptoms are the outcome of activity of nervous elements untouched by any pathological process'. Therefore, the argument runs, the pathological is a manifestation of some aspect of at least part of a normal mechanism. But returning to Gregory's (1961) analogy with a radio set this argument would indicate that the howling of a radio with a capacitor removed or damaged was simply an exaggeration of a normal part of the radio's ordinary behavioural repertoire.

In the more important sense this is clearly false; the howling dominates the radio's behaviour in a quite abnormal way, and is due to an oscillation which would not arise with the capacitor working. Similarly, spasticity of the limbs which is caused by certain types of brain damage, or tremor as in Parkinson's disease, can become so exaggerated as to dominate behaviour and indeed the sufferer's whole life, but not reveal anything profound about normal mechanisms. It might be argued that, in the sense that the howling radio set emits a loud sound, nothing but an exaggerated aspect of normal behaviour (making a sound) is being exhibited. But does this not trivialize the issue? Even more to the point is whether it reveals anything fundamental about how the radio set makes the howling sound, or indeed a sound of any sort.

The fact that certain behavioural potentialities can be exaggerated thus gives no easy insight into how either the normal or the exaggerated behaviour is produced. It is still behaviour needing to be explained and the chief result of the physiological intervention may not be to expose its workings but to draw attention to it.

The argument, therefore, amounts to the proposition that drawing of attention to a phenomenon may be important. Lorenz (1969) for instance seems to support this in claiming that the 'essentially pathological' discharge of patterns of behaviour *in vacuo*, when the normal eliciting circumstances were not present was the type of observation upon which ethology was founded. These species-specific behaviour patterns would not have been noticed or their independence of external co-ordinating stimuli understood except for such 'pathological' occurrences. Is it not, however, more than stretching a point to categorize such matters as pathological? Lorenz's attribution 'pathological' seems to be used in a different sense here. What he is talking about is the operation of perfectly normal mechanisms in what seem to be inappropriate environmental circumstances. This certainly is helpful in attracting the scientist's attention since the observations suggest unsuspected characteristics that normal mechanisms have. Visual illusions serve the same function, as Wittgenstein (1953) proposed, of making aspects of vision seem puzzling or surprising, so that we do not take the whole process of vision for granted.

The malfunction caused by a lesion is of a quite different kind. It too may well be puzzling and attract attention, but as in the case of the howling radio set, attention can be attracted to some feature which is scarcely part of normal behaviour at all. Indeed, much of our experience with broken down mechanisms indicate that quite often what is exaggerated is the trivial or at least the non-essential (cf. backfiring in cars, television pictures that fail to hold, radios where distortion occurs because of a battery running down, etc). To extend a typical Hughlings-Jackson argument a little, if higher functions are dependent on a rather delicate and subtle organization of 'higher' processes, then destroying that organization can only reveal 'lower', more disorganized behaviour.

Taking the problem to the computer again allows a better insight into why although a good theory of a mechanism allows us to understand a malfunction, studying the malfunction does not necessarily yield a theory of how the mechanism normally works. If one takes a small segment of program in a familiar scientific programming language such as ALGOL the oddity of exploding small bombs inside the computer to find out how it works, and the nature of the information that can be derived from similar techniques on the brain becomes clearer. Consider the following segment of program in the form of an ALGOL procedure for computing factorials for positive integers. The program is rather inefficient in terms of machine usage because it requires a lot of computer time repeatedly to enter procedures. Nevertheless, the example is fairly simple and illustrative.

```
integer procedure factorial (n);
integer n;
value n;
if n = 1 then factorial: = n else
factorial: = n * factorial (n-1);
```

Now in this section of program there are clearly some distinct and recognizable elements: the line, the word, algebraic symbols like =, and so on. Perhaps we could find out something of the program's behaviour by judiciously removing some of these. If one removed the third line for instance, then the amount of computing time might with some calls of this procedure be increased. Removal of the next line would lead to bizarre behaviour. The program would enter a continuous loop and fail to converge on a solution, though after a time the computer would output a message like 'INTEGER OVERFLOW', or run out of store. If one removed one of the smaller elements, say, the symbol ;, then the program would not run at all, but an error message would appear while the program was being compiled.

Clearly from this sort of evidence in whatever quantity it would be impossible to understand anything important about how the program works. Indeed for someone unversed in programming these 'behaviours' will already from my description be incomprehensible. We would simply collect a mass of quite striking pieces of 'abnormal' behaviour, perhaps get the impression that if we could understand them then they must tell us something about how the program works, and assert that at the very least we were collecting facts about the workings of this program which any theory purporting to explain it must finally take account of.

However, the situation is even worse than it seems. Not only are the data from such 'lesion' studies uninterpretable if one does not already understand the program, but these particular lesions were done under the most favourable possible conditions. They were done where the elements removed were in fact functional elements in the logical organization of the program, i.e. a line or statement in this program corresponds to a single functional operation. If we were making lesions in the computer, rather than its program, then these lesions need not correspond to functional entities in the logical structure. That is to say, there is no anatomically distinct part or parts of the computer, no circuit board, or bunch of wires, which correspond to these functional entities in the program. Thus if we remove some anatomically distinct part from the machine, this does not even carry the guarantee that the piece is functionally distinct.

The reason for this is somewhat as follows. ALGOL has signs such as := and - which relate expressions to one another in a language rather similar to mathematics. Thus for performing mathematical calculations like finding factorials the language and syntax used by the programmer merely has to define or state in formal terms what a factorial is. This definition is, of course, useless until it has been translated into computer instructions which actually operate the hardware. In a computer most information is represented as sequences of binary switches in either their 'on' or 'off' position. Bi-stable switches in particular positions in a sequence, in particular 'on' or 'off' states, determine whether a number is 12 or 13, whether a logical proposition is being asserted as true or false, what the address of some stored information is, and so forth. In the computer a 'lower level' program called a compiler accepts a specific 'higher level' ALGOL program and maps it onto a sequence of instructions to open and close particular binary switches. The sequences of 'on' and 'off' switches are a yet 'lower' level representation of the information.

Here one approaches the heart of the problem. The ALGOL language has a syntax and internal organization in a domain suitable for representing and expressing mathematics. The domain of machine code has a syntax suitable for organizing binary switching sequences. Mapping these languages from one domain to the other is a very complicated business, and there is no one-to-one or other simple correspondence between the elements of one language and the elements of the other. On different occasions when the program is run, different storage locations in the computer are likely to be used. Furthermore, though a particular part of the central processor always performs the operation of subtraction, which appears in ALGOL as a unique symbol, that particular piece of hardware also performs additions, and so on. Very few, if any, one-to-one correspondences exist between part of the ALGOL program and parts of the computer hardware. It follows that by paying attention to any one single piece of hardware by lesioning it or recording from it one will not be paying attention to a single structural (logical) element of the program.

Part of the explanation of how an ALGOL program works concerns the process of compilation just discussed. This process might possibly be hinted at by lesion experiments, since some lesions would prevent compilation being completed and an error message might appear. But even the notion of two separate processes, compiling and running, would simply be a confirmation of what one knew from other sources. In order to run the program at all, the operator would have to know (or have found) first how to do one thing (to compile) and then how to do something else (to run).

It seems clear that even at this level of explanation the lesion is inefficient at producing information which leads to understanding. In order to understand the piece of program for computing factorials one has to go about it in quite a different way. One has to understand what a factorial (the equivalent of some piece of behaviour) is, what significance the various elements of ALGOL have, and also to understand the rather difficult notion of recursion. In this concept the ALGOL compiler allows a function to be defined partly in terms of itself.

A quick description of how this ALGOL procedure works when called by the main program (which again for people lacking the conceptual schemata of programming may not be very clear) might be as follows. The first three lines are essentially headings and declarations allowing the computer to be able correctly to interpret the symbol n. The next line says that if n, the variable for which the factorial is to be found, is one, then the procedure returns the value n which in this case would be 1 as the result (i.e. the value of n's factorial). However, if the original n is larger than 1 the last line says that the value of the factorial is n times the value of the factorial of n-1. This line, therefore, calls the factorial procedure again, but now enters it with a value of n which is one less than before. The procedure will indeed go on calling itself, i.e. re-entering the same procedure making n less by 1 each time until by continually doing n-1, it gets to a value where n is 1, when the process will terminate. Next the computer, as it were, backs up through the series starting with n = 1, and putting in actual values for n and factorial (n-1) at each stage. For instance, for n = 2 the sequence will have terminated by finding that 2-1 is 1, and calling the procedure with that value (1) for n, and returning the result 1. It can now calculate that factorial 2 is n times factorial (n-1) which is $2 \times 1 = 2$. The program solves factorial 3 by adding an extra stage, factorial 4 by another stage, and so on, up to whatever value of n was in the original call of the procedure.

Though this may all seem very laborious and possibly opaque, recursion is an important concept in both computing and in language. It is usually only understood thoroughly after some weeks of writing programs oneself which contain recursive operations. This example illustrates that in order to understand the structure, symbols and arrangement of the program we have to have a well developed and not necessarily simple theory of schema of how the program works. Without such a theory we could not make sense of it. (Some might say it is even pretty difficult with such a theory.) In this context it seems odd to suppose that we could confront a structure as organizationally complex as the brain and try to understand it simply by looking, let alone by poking it about or chopping bits off.

To say that we cannot understand a system without, from the beginning, having some theory (and even experience) about how it works seems like a counsel of despair. It is the theory of how it works that we want as an end product and it is precisely what we do not have at the beginning. This is, however, less a counsel of despair than a recognition of how human cognition and understanding seem to work. What it seems to call for in brain research are fewer uninterpretable observations of the consequences of manipulating brain tissue, and more inventions and experience of how interesting kinds of behaviour could be produced. Without having some theory of how a factorial could be calculated at all, it is difficult to see how we could discover how some system (brain or computer) in particular does it.

The above arguments do not, of course, mean that brain lesions cannot disclose important and unsuspected properties of the brain. Rather I want to suggest that they are inappropriate vehicles for asking the question of how a mechanism works. A much more appropriate target for the technique is the investigation of the brain's resistance to damage: the surprising fact that the brain continues to go on working rather well despite enormous devastation of its parts, and despite other kinds of disruptive noise. This aspect is an apt target for the lesion technique. Clearly if the brain does continue to work quite well despite extensive damage or loss of any individual components, then this property sets it apart from almost every type of physical device with which we are familiar, in which damage to a single component typically makes the whole device defective or useless. One way of attacking this matter is to produce experimental brain lesions in order to investigate both the limits and nature of this remarkable property wherein the whole is more reliable than any of its parts, and the important work begun by Lashley on this problem will be discussed in a later chapter.

A second use for the lesion is to isolate parts of the brain in the hope that the properties of these parts will be simpler than that of the whole. In a sense the neurophysiological study of a single nerve cell involves this kind of manipulation. Equally clearly the same principle is involved in studying an isolated ganglion in an invertebrate, an isolated retina, or an animal with only the spinal cord functioning and connected to the muscles. Particularly if the isolated part has some functional autonomy and is capable of giving rise to components of the behaviour of the whole organism it is entirely appropriate to suppose that studying the part may allow a simplification so that some mechanisms producing its behaviour can be more easily understood. In just the same way isolation of the teletypewriter of a computer from the main machine might be a valuable step towards investigating the particular properties of the teletypewriter. Removing all but one of its peripheral devices from a computer might be another good move, but in each case it is probably important that some normal communication channels remain. Thus though it is rather clear that study of the behaviour of animals with only the spinal cord working has led to important understanding of the nature of behaviour (e.g. Sherrington, 1906), it is by no means as clear that the study of the isolated slab of cortex (e.g. Burns, 1958) has the same kinds of potentiality for understanding how behaviour is produced, since we do not know how to communicate with it in a way that the cortex is usually communicated with, nor can we understand the significance of its responses.

This does not necessarily mean that the isolated cortical slab is not useful in the physiological sense for studying properties of isolated neural networks. However, one should be aware that the notion of simplifying a mechanism by removing some of its parts easily topples into the reductionist fallacy. If the behaviour of a whole were deducible simply from the properties of its parts, then tackling the parts one at a time clearly would make the task easier. But it is the fact of properties derived not from the parts themselves but principally from complex interactions between parts (as in a language structure, or presumably as in the brain) that makes the idea that an anatomical lesion necessarily results in the simplification of deleting a specific function from the behavioural repertoire so implausible.

A somewhat different argument that the problems of the brain can be simplified by surgery or other direct manipulations is that almost any insult we can offer to brain tissue in the form of lesion, stimulation, or pharmacological manipulation that allows some behaviour to be produced will cause some kind of disruption. The cerebral manipulation is likely to affect some aspects of behaviour more than others, and the whole imponderable complex of behaviour might then start to crack apart at its seams.

It does seem to be a logical conclusion that if a lesion does leave an animal with one aspect of behaviour affected and another not, the mechanisms generating the two aspects must be in some respect different. If, for instance, a lesion can be made that affects acquisition of some learned response, but does not affect extinction, and a different lesion has the opposite effect of affecting extinction but not acquisition, a state of affairs called double dissociation is produced. This would be evidence that acquisition and extinction were in at least one (albeit unknown) respect different processes and not, as has been assumed in some learning theories, the same. There are other examples of this double dissociation technique which have given support to the conceptual separation of defferent aspects of behaviour. For instance, in Schneider's (1969) experiments ablation of the visual cortex of the hamster leads to loss of pattern vision but not of visual direction finding; removal of the superior colliculus abolishes the animal's visual directional sense but apparently leaves intact its pattern vision.

In so far as some particular parts of the brain seem to be more particularly concerned with one aspect of behaviour than another, in the way that the retina, the optic nerves and tracts, the superior colliculus and the lateral geniculate body and the striate area seem to be particularly (though probably not exclusively) concerned with vision, some important knowledge has been gained. But one should beware of the extension of the argument that because behaviour can be seen as having different aspects, memory, attention, expectancy, and so on, that behaviour can be regarded as composed of these aspects like so many ingredients mixed together in a fruit cake. One should also note that the anatomical impressions that one part is concerned principally with this and another part with that are not of any great value in themselves.

Lashley wrote the passage about textbook anatomy, which is one of the three with which this book started in 1930. 'The chapter on the nervous system seems to provide an excuse for pictures in an otherwise dry and monotonous text. That it has any other function is not clear.' The situation is not much improved today. In so far as the situation has improved, as for instance, in analysis of the workings of the retina, it is due to relatively well developed theories of how certain features of behaviour (e.g. aspects of colour vision) might be produced (e.g. in Helmholtz's (1860) and Hering's (1878) theories), and allowing interpretation of physiological experiments to be guided by these theories, and directed towards particular retinal structures by anatomical knowledge. The anatomical knowledge and psychological theory thus have to be exploited by the physiological techniques to give the physiology meaning.

For the most part, although the so called functional anatomy (that this bit of the brain is concerned with that aspect of behaviour) still serves principally the purpose that Lashley pointed out of providing pictures for textbooks.

One implication of the foregoing argument is that techniques like lesioning and electrical stimulation of the brain should be regarded principally as attempts to identify components of behaviour and not at all as a means of localizing the functional components of the brain. Until now, however, it is not clear that identification of behavioural components and formulation of fruitful theoretical constructs on the basis of purely behavioural data has had to await interpretation of behavioural fragmentation by physiological manipulation. Often indeed until operational definitions of various behavioural components are produced, the physiological dissociation would again not be interpretable. In human memory the distinction between short and long term verbal memory, and means for identifying and measuring each aspect, were needed in order that these same means could be used in confirming a distinction between two categories of remembering on the grounds of their independent existence in different types of clinical amnesia caused by brain damage (Baddeley and Warrington, 1970; Shallice and Warrington, 1970). The distinction, though reified by the physiological 'lesions', was not made on the basis of such data.

The foregoing arguments have concerned mainly the lesion technique and its limitations as a means for revealing how brain mechanisms work. The techniques of direct stimulation of the brain clearly suffer from the same kinds of drawbacks. That is to say, production of some piece of behaviour by an electrical or chemical stimulus does not reveal how the behaviour is produced. The logical pitfalls may be glimpsed by working through the example of the computer program again, but now initiating the program at any arbitrary point. Again, bizarre, attention provoking and strange behaviour will be produced. But it is either behaviour which is well organized so that we have merely learned that it can be provoked artificially; or it is odd in some way. In either case we are no nearer to understanding how the mechanisms work.

In summary, the kinds of conclusions that may be drawn from lesion and stimulation research are as follows.

A The techniques give some indication of which areas of the brain are involved in which aspects of behaviour. This may be useful for later physiological research in that it directs attention to certain areas. The identification of brain regions with aspects of behaviour does not, however, constitute an explanation of how the behaviour is produced.

B Lesions reveal the important fact that the brain often continues working coherently and adaptively despite extensive damage to its parts, and that in many instances well organized behaviour is not dependent on particular components.

C Isolation of parts of the brain that are autonomously capable of co-ordinated behaviour may under some, but not all circumstances, present a simplified task for behavioural analysis.

D Any direct manipulation of brain tissue may cause a disruption of behaviour, and if different aspects of behaviour are differentially affected, as well as drawing attention to them, this indicates that these aspects are separable logically, and do not arise from exactly the same mechanism.

Thus although lesions and stimulation very directly affect brain tissue, and allow some conclusions to be drawn one cannot conclude that they reveal the workings of that tissue, any more than similar interventions in a computer would reveal how the machine played chess, solved an equation, or calculated factorials. Indeed, in general, in so far as behaviour produced by a direct brain manipulation is different from normal, the difference seems to be rather a poor guide to how either the normal or the pathological behaviour is produced. If the object of brain research is to give an account of how neural operations generate behaviour, then changing the nature of behaviour by making it pathological essentially creates a new species, and may leave the original task untouched. If the behaviour that remains is simplified, then this task of analysis may be made easier but the simplified behaviour may be distorted, or even comparatively trivial.

MICRO-ELECTRODE RECORDING

If interpretation of results in physiological psychology is beset with difficulties, this is also true in neurophysiology. The favourite neurophysiological technique at present is that of micro-electrode recordings of single cell activity, usually, though no longer exclusively, in anaesthetized animals. Information has been obtained about the types of stimuli to which cells can specifically respond, e.g. by a change in their mean firing rate. For example, it seems that the brain is able to detect in visual patterns the presence of small line-segments (Hubel and Wiesel, 1959) and to detect movement (Barlow and Hill, 1963) as a basic attribute of a stimulus. Single cells also seem capable of responding specifically to the spatial frequency of a pattern (Campbell, Cooper and Enroth-Cugell, 1969), to retinal disparity (Barlow, Blakemore and Pettigrew, 1967), novelty (Horn and Hill, 1964) and so on. The easy conclusion to draw from this type of result is that firing of these cells in response to a stimulus with some property constitutes recognition by the organism, of that aspect of the stimulus.

However, even when neurones responding to rather complex arrangements are discovered, such as for instance Gross *et al*'s (1972) neurones in a monkey which apparently are specifically responsive to the shape of a primate hand, this tells us simply that the brain has the means for differentiating this aspect of the visual world, from other aspects; information which we can also get by behavioural means. Without other data it does not tell us what role in analysing the visual image that cell plays. Nor does it tell us the mechanism by which the cell was enabled to respond so specifically.

The reason why single unit recording in the mammalian visual system has been so remarkably successful is not that this technique alone has established our present understanding of the physiology of vision, but that this method provides data which can be understood because of an already well articulated psychological understanding of vision. Some fundamental processes such as colour analysis, lateral inhibition, movement detection and so forth, though now relatively well understood in terms of neurone interactions, would probably not be understood if single unit data had been all that were available.

Many of the results, moreover, are only understood now in terms of a questionable theory of stimulus classification, to be discussed in the next chapter. Even in the case of Hubel and Wiesel's (1959) famous finding of line segment detectors in the cat's cortex, these data or their possible extensions do not in themselves allow us to understand pattern recognition. Nor is it even clear within physiological terms what these units do. They change their firing rate similarly for a change of line orientation, or length, or position, or disparity or spatial frequency. So what can it be said that one of these neurones is detecting? The change of firing rate is in itself ambiguous. This kind of neurophysiological information, in order to be useful, has to be interpretable, and this state has yet to be reached. Only by reference of the physiological data to some fairly comprehensive schema or theory which can given an account of the properties of vision can we create some better idea of what role feature detecting elements might actually play (see chapter 7 for one such attempt).

BRAIN RESEARCH AND THEORY

It seems then that any anatomical or physiological datum can only be interpreted by viewing that datum in the light of some theory; just as in the perception process itself a datum such as a line segment can only be interpreted within the context of other data, and of the brain's representational structure. In particular, we are short of psychological theories which spell out how behaviour and mental processes could conceivably be produced. Therefore, in trying to understand behaviour in terms of the workings of the brain the different fields of study — anatomy, biophysics, neurophysiology, physiological psychology, and psychology — should really be treated as different but inter-dependent techniques at different levels within the field of brain research, each informed by specifications of required behaviour at the next higher level, and by understanding of the components at the lower level. Most of all, they would be informed by a rich repertoire of conceptual schemata capable of describing how behaviour at that level of analysis could be produced.

It might have been imagined that biological brains would have been very difficult to do experiments on. Almost the reverse has turned out to be true. If fact, it is no more difficult to do experiments on the brain than to do experiments in chemistry. Indeed, experiments multiply with extraordinary fecundity, especially experiments on previous methods and on previous experiments. The result is a very large amount of data on particularities of brains and behaviour, but not necessarily much that is cumulative or enlightening about the larger problems.

Scientific discoveries seem to be of two kinds. There are some processes which before the understanding of some essential point seem mysterious: we do not know how an event occurs. When somebody finds out the way in which it happens, it might even be surprising, but once we can see how it is done, it becomes less interesting. In a second type of discovery the process which has been discovered remains interesting even after it is understood. The mechanism may itself reflect some fundamental principle of a larger problem, and the way in which the process occurs is not arbitrary. The mechanism of natural selection is one such discovery not merely because it has become central to biological thinking. The same type of thing obtains in very much smaller more specialized areas. The function of the auditory ossicles in matching the acoustic impedence of air to that of water is an instance (Helmholtz, 1862). If one defines the problem correctly it would scarcely have been done otherwise. It is thus a very satisfying example of an appropriate mechanism.

The difficulty with brain research is that there seem to be relatively few discoveries of this second type. More typically it has been found that some piece of brain is involved in this process rather than that one. Or that behaviour involves this piece of brain more than that piece. Such discoveries do not embody the essence of what is brainlike, and tend, unless they become involved in some new experimental method, to lose interest soon after they are made.

What might be more productive would be concentration on those problems that are essentially and distinctively brain-like, rather than on less fundamental issues. Enquiring into what examples of such processes might be, we can return to Craik (1943). He suggested that the brain can generate intelligent behaviour because it parallels relationships of time and space between external events in an internal model. This is, of course, only one way of looking at the problem but it seems possible that this is at least one of the essentially brainlike processes, and that by investigating and understanding it some important principles by which intelligent behaviour is generated might be discovered.

One difficulty is in deciding what research one should do. Craik suggested that experiments in which animals or people re-learned artificially disordered relationships in the external world, could provide evidence about how the brain model adapts to parallel the environment. Clearly more than this is needed to find out whether the principle of the brain containing a model of the world is a fruitful and enlightening one. We would need to show as a minimum that some range of problems was more easily understood along these than along any other lines. More powerfully we would need to demonstrate that some problems could not be tackled without invoking, for instance, the principle of an internally modelled environment.

One simple example of this is provided by the problem of motivated behaviour in animals. Until about thirty years ago the whole issue of purposeful behaviour seemed mysterious. It was obscured by vitalism, and the very concept of purposefulness was denounced as 'teleological'. The difficulty was that people could not see how an event in the future (a desired effect) could influence processes in the present, when causality works in exactly the opposite temporal sequence. We understand now that this is possible precisely because desired events in the future can be symbolically represented in the brain, and behaviour can be generated by means of a comparison between the symbolic desired state and a measurement of the present actual state. The problem can be understood by proposing that the brain has an internal representation of the desired future state, but not otherwise. A formal basis for these arguments is now contained in control theory, and its specific application to one form of motivated behaviour, i.e. thirst (e.g. Oatley, 1970) has provided a detailed understanding of some of the mechanisms involved. Furthermore, in order to understand other aspects of motivated behaviour it is enlightening to formulate the problem in terms of the animal operating with a model in which are manipulated symbolic representations of processes important to the animal in both its internal and external environments.

The point is that with the concepts and theoretical framework of feedback control systems and control theory we can think about problems such as homeostasis and certain types of motivated behaviour productively. Without such concepts we can scarcely think about the problem at all, we do not know what observations are important, and the interpretation of those that are made is difficult.

What seems necessary is that we invent what Chomsky (1965) has called competence models for behaviour: mechanisms that conceivably could undertake tasks central to animals' and peoples' tasks of living successfully in their environments. For instance, we might be able to obtain insight into the brain's model of the world by inspecting and characterizing those aspects of the environment with which we have commerce, and which, therefore, the brain has to represent in some way. Although such a characterization, which might include some features of events relevant to the animal's life in its environment, is an important first step, this characterization is unlikely to be exactly the same as that used by the brain. A characterization in terms of a competence model might be chosen for formal simplicity, that of the brain might be organized in quite other ways. Experimentation can be directed by our model of how some process might be achieved at all, and our understanding refined by the mismatches between what that model can generate, and actual behaviour.

This, of course, is a statement of the method of hypothesis and experimental disconfirmation. The reason for restating it here is that brain research continues in an atmosphere of extraordinarily impoverished theory. It even occasionally carries the assumption that one can make direct observations of facts of the brain, or of behaviour untrammelled by theory. In this chapter I hope to have given some indication that the typical kinds of observations that are made are not as revealingly direct as they might seem. In the next chapter I shall argue that there is a theory which permeates brain research, sometimes explicitly and, despite denials, sometimes implicitly. Given that our scientific (and indeed any other cognitive) activity is theory directed, our progress is hampered by the inadequacy of theoretical structure.

4 *Theories of brain function*

REQUIREMENTS FOR THEORIES OF BEHAVIOUR

It is fair to set up two criteria for assessing theories (particularly 'formal' theories) for which the claim is made that they in some way explain behaviour. First, an adequate theory must be capable of producing in a specified way something which corresponds to at least some aspect of behaviour. A small boy on being offered a model car would be direly disappointed on being given something made of clay with wheels that did not even go round. Yet we are offered theories of behaviour which are often even more disappointing: equivalent to a series of tickets joined together with string, and with the tickets bearing legends that might for a model car be 'direction system', 'backfiring inhibitor' and so on. Clearly, many theoretical attempts have no mechanism, no formal set of rules, no criteria, indeed no operations capable of producing anything, let alone events corresponding to behaviour.

A second requirement for a theory to be taken seriously is that it should itself display principles that make the behaviour possible. For instance, if someone said that he or she had an explanation of language embodied in a humanoid mechanism, and this turned out to be a doll which produced pre-recorded sentences, in a pseudo-random order when a string in the doll's back was pulled to wind the record mechanism, nobody would be impressed. Yet the mechanism produces some recognizable behaviour by its own workings. The inadequacy here, of course, is that no principles of how meaningful linguistic utterances are constructed is deployed in the mechanism. The behaviour is simply a copy of behaviour produced by a person.

A mechanism, computer program, or formal statement of the rules in a theory must, therefore, be able itself to produce behaviour of a non-trivial kind by means of its own operations, without human judgments having to be applied (it may be the nature of these judgments we wish to explain). Being able to emit behaviour sequences which are just copies of human behaviour, or which are already specified by the designer, is not enough.

Of course, the question of what one means by principles making behaviour or mental processes possible is a difficult one. It is often true that one thinks one has grasped some such principle, and then on applying it in various situations begins to glimpse its inadequacy. Indeed, this ingredient of disconfirmation or refutation as Popper (1963) would call it is an essential one in the growth of theories, i.e. understandings of important principles.

Being able to grasp exactly where and how some particular theory falls short is part of the process of enlarging our understanding. Unsatisfying though it may seem, many of our more important conclusions about the brain so far have been of this kind: the demonstration that existing hypotheses do not reach far enough. This state of affairs is only disappointing at first sight. With a second look what we have as a result of the many demonstrations in the literature of how brain mechanisms cannot possibly work is a growing set of criteria that adequate explanations of behaviour must meet; a growing awareness of the subtlety and intricacy of behaviour, and of what the important (non-trivial) principles underlying behaviour and mental processes might be.

Even more important is that in the failures or mistakes a theory makes are often the clues to the means of improvement. Just as in our ordinary lives we learn best by our mistakes, applying our always incomplete theories about how to live to an uncompromising world, often failing, and occasionally thereby improving our understanding, so a scientific theory can grow when it fails in some well structured way. The difficulty, of course, both in ordinary life and in the pursuit of scientific understanding, is the temptation of self justification, and the inability to recognize the mistake or disconfirmation. If it is recognized, changing the theory (a difficult and exacting matter) may or may not be possible within the available resources, intellectual or otherwise. I hope to be able to show how the currently held (though not always explicitly stated) theory of brain mechanisms has been disconfirmed in a variety of ways and that we are now in the fortunate position of having better theories to move to.

As it happens there seem as yet to have been only a few basic types of explanation of behaviour that can be said to qualify as theories, in that models representing these theories can themselves actually produce behaviour of some kind. Thus there is not a great deal of ground to cover, and understanding what these theories can and cannot explain is fundamental. Indeed, it seems to be the case that one basic theory, that of the reflex, or stimulus and response, pervades a great deal of thinking both in psychology and in the physiology of brains. One sees it in the continuous use of the words like stimulus, reponse and connection (or association) in talking about brains, behaviour and mental processes. Despite possible denials by the users, these terms are not facts, but theory laden concepts, and concepts are part of understanding. What then are the characteristics of reflex theory, explicit or implicit?

REFLEX THEORY: STIMULUS → RESPONSE

We need go no further in looking for a succinct statement of the reflex theory of brain mechanism than the writings of Descartes (1664, 1667), who was not only the first to propose this hypothesis, but the first to propose any kind of formalizable theory of mechanism for the brain. Moreover, one cannot do better in describing this theory than to quote directly from Descartes. First here is Descartes' analogy with automatically operated statues in the gardens of the Royal Palace at Saint-Germain.

> The external objects that by their presence alone act upon the sensory organs ... are like strangers who entering into one of the grottos of these fountains ... cannot enter without stepping on certain tiles so placed that, for instance if they approach a bathing Diana they will cause her to hide in the rushes; and if they go in pursuit of her, they will cause Neptune to approach menacingly with his trident; or if they go to one side they will cause a sea monster to appear and spew water in their faces, or similar things according to the whim of the engineers who made them. Finally there is a reasoning soul in this machine (the body); it has its principal site in the brain where it is like the fountaineer who must be at the reservoir, whither all the pipes of these machines are extended, when he wishes to start, stop or in some way alter their actions.

Next Descartes describes how these principles are applied to a human withdrawal reflex (letters refer to fig. 4.1);

> As for example if the fire A is near the foot B the particles of this fire which as you know move with great rapidity, have the power to move the area of skin which they touch; and in this way drawing the little thread that you see attached there, at the same instant they open the entrance of the pore d, e, at which this little thread terminates ... Now the entrance to the pore or little conduit d, e, being thus opened the animal spirits in the cavity F enter within and are carried by it partly into the muscles that serve to withdraw this foot from the fire, partly into these that serve to turn the eyes and the head to look at it, and partly into those that serve to advance the hands and to bend the whole body to protect it.

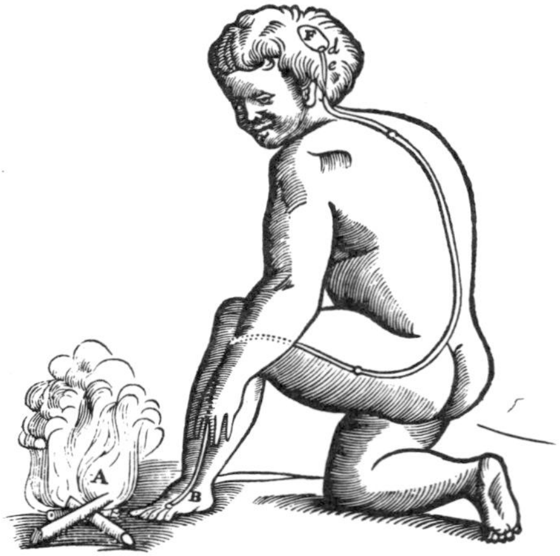

Figure 4.1 Descartes' (1664) illustration the reflex.

Basically therefore Descartes viewed the ventricles in the brain as a reservoir into which the heart had pumped up a head of fluid (animal spirits). The little strings opened valves, and thereby this fluid could be let into tubes to inflate those muscles which were appropriate to the particular stimulus. Summarizing the mechanisms of sensory nerves as involving the pulling of little threads, and of motor nerves as being tubular conductors of fluid to the muscles Descartes writes:

> There are three things to be considered in the nerves: ... their medulla or internal substance is extended in the form of little threads from the brain; ... then that the membranes which surround them and which are continuous with the one that envelops the brain are composed of little tubes in which these fine little threads are enclosed; and finally that the animal spirits that are carried in these same tubes from the brain to the muscles explain why the threads are quite free and so plentiful, so that the least thing which moves the part of the body or extremity to which one of them is attached, in the same way causes movement in the part of the brain from which it comes; just as when one end of a cord is pulled the other end moves.

The way in which the fluid as well as inflating muscles serves to lubricate the threads is a very nice touch.

Next, Descartes enlarges upon his notion of a response.

> Now as these spirits thus enter into the cavity of the brain so they pass from there into the pores of its substance, and from these pores into the nerves; where as they enter ... they have the power to change the shape of the muscles in which the nerves are inserted and by this means to cause motions in all the parts. Just as you may have seen that the power of moving water travelling from its source is alone sufficient to move the machines in the grottos and fountains in our king's gardens according to the various arrangements of the pipes conducting it, even causing these machines to play several instruments or to pronounce several words.

> No single movement can take place either in the bodies of animals or in ours if these bodies do not have in them all the organs and instruments by means of which these same movements could also be accomplished by a machine...

> Among the movements that take place in our bodies there are some that do not at all depend upon the mind, such as the beating of the heart, the digestion of food, nutrition, respiration of those who are asleep and even of those who are awake, walking, singing and other similar actions when they take place without the mind thinking of them. When those who fall from a height thrust their hands to protect

> their heads, it is not on the advice of reason that they perform this action, and it does not depend upon their mind, but only upon their senses which, being aware of the present danger ... cause the animal spirit to pass from there (the brain) into the nerves in the fashion that is required, to produce the movement immediately.

Finally a way in which such a mechanism may accommodate learning is proposed (cit Lashley, 1950)

> When the mind wills to recall something, this volition causes the little (pineal) gland, by inclining successively to different sides, to impel the animal spirits toward different parts of the brain, until they come upon that part where the traces are left of the thing which it wishes to remember; for these traces are nothing else than the circumstance that the pores of the brain through which the spirits have already taken their course on presentation of the object, have thereby acquired a greater facility than the rest to be opened again the same way by the spirits which come to them; so that these spirits coming upon the pores enter therein more readily than the others.

There is nothing outdated about these notions; as Lashley (1950) remarked about the last of these passages 'Descartes' theory has a remarkably modern sound. Substitute nerve impulse for animal spirits, synapse for pore'. Indeed, major achievements of neurophysiology and neural biophysics have been precisely those of discovering the electro-chemical equivalents of strings and tubes for communication over long distances, and the mechanism of synaptic valves that allow switching of signals.

One important point is now clear. Both information transmission and logical operations are independent of the means by which they are performed. A system of strings, valves and hydraulics may be clumsier, certainly slower and probably less reliable over many operations than, say, an electronic system, but there need be no difference in principle between the way a switching operation could be arranged to operate, say, a statue, and a more modern machine such as an automatically activated supermarket door, when some particular event occurs. The same information, or logical operations, could be handled by many types of system, including the electro-chemico-mechanical system of nerves and muscles.

Descartes' theory has a number of features which are worth examining in detail in order to determine the light they shed on the nature of behaviour.

A MECHANISM OF LOGICAL OPERATIONS THAT DOES PRODUCE BEHAVIOUR

Descartes' use of the analogy with hydraulically actuated garden statues demonstrates unequivocably how a mechanism of the kind he describes could produce behaviour. It also demonstrates how the beginning of our understanding of the brain requires the comparison with a more familiar 'physical' system. It seems minimally that understanding of a common principle necessitates comparisons of at least two different examples.

Equally important is the fact that the mechanism works by performing logical operations on input information: the function of the valves (pores) is to perform the operation 'if stimulus S_1 occurs then release response R_1'.

Although there have been currents within the general literature of reflexology that have described the mechanism as being that of reflecting energy from the environment to drive the responses of the musculature, this was not any part of Descartes' proposal. His mechanisms were entirely informational; the energy source for the movement being quite properly kept separate and consisting of the potential energy of the head of fluid that had been pumped up into the ventricular reservoirs in the brain.

In many ways these major aspects of Descartes' account — his argument that behaviour which after all does consist of movements, could only be accomplished via the agency of some kind of machine, that the type of machine required is one that also has means of communicating information, that it works by elementary switching operations, and that the movements produced are appropriate to external events — are the most important of his theory. For these aspects at least we have as yet no plausible alternative. Furthermore, since machines based on logical (switching) operations, can perform some behaviour appropriate to environmental events, maybe machines more sophisticated than those envisaged by Descartes but still using logical operations as a basis, might be able to encroach upon the area he reserved for the 'reasoning mind'. By his own argument this too must involve machinery since it too has to perform movements, namely, the pineal gland inclining to one or other side to open pores. It is clear too that if the brain does work by performing elementary logical operations, then just as Descartes used hydraulic machines of his day as analogies, we can produce behaviour using artificial machines that can also carry out logical operations. The question of whether the activities of nerve cells that we do understand are correctly understood as means for performing logical switching operations is of fundamental importance. If this is the role of nerve cells, then sequences of such logical operations will underly behaviour either where it is determined innately ('by the whim of the engineers who made them') or by learning. However, it is the arrangement of switching operations that specifies the behaviour.

The next aspect of Descartes' theory of interest is the implicit proposition that not all behaviour and mental processes are explicable in terms of reflex connections. Some behaviour is created by the reasoning mind. This, of course, is the feature of his theory which has attracted the most attention, in that from it has developed the doctrine of mind-body dualism. Making suitable allowance for possible religious 'impediments' to understanding, Descartes' idea of the reasoning mind or soul might simply be taken as the statement that whereas some aspects of behaviour seem explicable in terms of reflex responses, others do not. It does indeed seem difficult to capture the essence of reasoning within the framework of reflexes and if Descartes claimed mind for man and denied it to animals, this is a distinction which need not have overtones of either religion or vitalism. This same point has been pressed with some force by Chomsky (1968) who also observed the parallel with Descartes in his claims of distinctively human linguistic capacities not explicable in terms of reflex mechanisms, and basic to mind. However, this need not mean that logical processes of a non-reflex kind would not be capable of producing rational thought.

Finally, there is the aspect of Descartes' theory that is most evident in the concepts of modern neurophysiology and psychology, the idea that there are objectively definable stimuli which the nervous system is constructed to detect and that similarly there are objectively definable responses which the nervous system can produce. With behaviour defined in these terms the job of brain research would presumably be to discover what stimuli there were, and how they are detected, and how they are connected to responses by the brain.

The following three sections are discussions of how reflex ideas, notions of stimulus, connection, and response permeate brain research, in some areas where the attempt to relate brain mechanisms to behaviour currently takes place, namely visual physiology, the problem of learning, and notions of levels of function in the brain.

The search for the adequate stimulus

The chances are that if one confronted research workers in neurophysiology, or experimental psychology, with the notion that our ideas about how the brain works still depend heavily on the theory of the reflex as put forward by Descartes, they would protest. However, a typical neurophysiologist might argue that he was trying to understand the capacity of neuronal networks to detect their adequate stimuli. Moreover a psychologist might say that we have dispensed with reflex theory long ago, and perhaps point to a loss of interest in subjects associated with behaviourism and a current interest in cognitive psychology. But if one looks at the book which is usually identified as heralding this new interest, Neisser's *Cognitive Psychology* (1967), one finds that in defining what is meant by this Neisser says that his book might have been called *Stimulus Information and its Vicissitudes*. And indeed, this alternative title captures very well the flavour of much cognitive psychology.

There is, in other words, by neurophysiologists and psychologists an easy acceptance of the concept 'stimulus'. So much so that it has become an almost unquestioned assumption that 'stimulus' is a perfectly straightforward unbiased descriptive term. Yet it is not. It is a theoretical term which carries a great deal of meaning, and in using it we are thinking, partly at least, within the conceptual framework of reflex or stimulus-response theory.

In Descartes' scheme the stimulus is the event in the environment that triggers the reflex movement: the fire that promotes withdrawal of the foot or the danger that makes one blink. Or is it? Perhaps it is the movement of the skin that pulls the string that opens the pore to let the animal spirits inflate a muscle. Herein lies the difficulty. Danger and excitation of a receptor are not the same. To use the same word 'stimulus' for both may obscure a wide gap in understanding.

The term stimulus is used in physiology in quite a general way to mean the immediate cause of excitation in any excitable tissue. Thus a sufficiently large electral current passed through the membrane of an axon will stimulate it, i.e. initiate a nerve impulse. Light will stimulate a photoreceptor, acetyle choline will stimulate a contraction in a denervated muscle, a train of electrical impulses applied to the precentral gyrus of the mammalian brain will stimulate movements.

The term 'stimulus' was discussed by Sherrington (1906) in the context of reflex arcs. 'Stimuli are', he observed, 'changes in the environment which impart energy to the organism.' But this energy is not funnelled through the organism to drive the response. Sherrington followed Descartes in arguing that stimulus energy acts as a trigger to release energy that the organism sets free. He described a simple reflex arc as consisting of receptor, conduction path, and effector. A reflex is elicited by stimulating the receptor. Within the terms of the mechanism the response might also be elicited by stimulating the sensory nerve itself, in the same way as the axons of the ulnar nerve can be stimulated by banging the elbow and giving rise to sensations in the fingers (the 'funny bone' effect). But some reflexes can only easily be elicited by stimulation of receptors. The function of the receptor, therefore, (argued Sherrington) is 'to lower the threshold of excitability of the (reflex) arc for one kind of stimulus and heighten it for all others'.

Thus Sherrington argued that whereas energy applied to the nerve itself might be unsuccessful in eliciting the response, a particular and appropriate form of energy applied to a particular part of the receptor surface would operate the reflex arc, because the receptors had become fitted by evolutionary adaptation to receive just that kind of energy, e.g. light, mechanical force etc. For an event to which a receptor was specially adapted, Sherrington coined the term 'adequate stimulus'. Electricity though it does stimulate receptors and other nerve cells quite easily is not usually defined as an adequate stimulus since electrical stimuli are not common in the natural environment and there has been little chance for organisms to evolve receptors appropriate to them. The receptor by its position on the body surface, and its selective excitability, is the important determinant of the specificity of reflexes since a given reflex will only be elicited by given types of energy applied to particular receptors in a certain position.

Sherrington's notion of the adequate stimulus has become one of the most important concepts in modern neurophysiology. With the discoveries by Hubel and Weisel (1959) and Lettvin, Matturana, McCulloch and Pitts (1959) that single cells of vertebrate sensory systems changed their firing rate in response to stimuli which were not just changes in light intensity on photo-receptors, but (respectively) straight line segments and even small flying bugs, the idea of the adequate stimulus entered a new phase. Sensory systems rather than just receptors, by being able to classify not just different types of stimulus energy but different types of stimulus pattern, might be able to bridge the gap between the event in the environment and the specific neural excitation: to make the connection between the danger of falling and the little strings that open the correct pores in the brain so that one extends one's hands in front of one.

If sensory systems were found to be able to classify environmental patterns in this way, this single capacity might allow a rigorous explanation of all sorts of complex behaviour on the basis of the reflex. A representative holder of this viewpoint is Horridge, who is the author of a widely respected monograph on interneurones (1968) and writer of review articles about neural integration (e.g. 1973). Within the context of a reflex theory clearly neural units must act to connect stimuli to responses. According to Horridge (1968) this occurs because (a) all interneurones (i.e. neurones which are connected only to other neurones) 'are units of pattern recognition'. Their responses 'are explicable as the consequence of particular patterns of summation and inhibition of earlier order neurones that impinge upon them'. Hence from the output of the receptor array onwards are banks of interneurones. Each will fire if the quantity of excitation arriving on its post-synaptic surfaces summates to outweigh inhibition and reach threshold. By virtue of the particular excitatory and inhibitory connections, therefore, each cell fires to some particular pattern of neural activity at the previous stage. Receptors are different in that by and large they respond only to single parameters of environmental stimulation, that is intensity and the like. Thus following the paths of impulses through the nervous system the outputs from any stage represent particular classifications of patterns that have been made, and the classifications are identified by the brain precisely by the activity of particular interneurones. The further from the receptor surface, the more abstract (presumably) the pattern class can conceivably be. Most interneurone responses cause no behaviour but finally one pattern will cause excitation above threshold at the final interneurone stage, and this will give rise to the behavioural response.

Environmental events of significance to the animal are thus detected. Then in so far as a particular event gives rise to an identifiable pattern of receptor stimulation, the neurone or neurones whose activities represent the classification evoke the appropriate choice of response from a finite repertoire of movements which are specifically adapted to the animal's mode of life. On this view learning is a matter of altering patterns of functional connectivity, according to principles of reinforcement or otherwise, so that new pattern classifications or new connections to response networks may be formed.

The major problem of explaining behaviour on this view, therefore, is essentially that of discovering what particular patterns of excitatory and inhibitory connections are made by neurones, and how these patterns of connection allow perhaps rather abstract features of the stimulus array to be classified successfully. Furthermore, the methodology of research that this suggests is fairly straightforward. First establish what patterns in the environment might be important in the life of the particular animal. Then record from interneurones while exposing them to these patterns, or components of these patterns. When neurones specifically responsive to the patterns presented have been found, the neurones will need to be identified and their connection traced: a Gargantuan task, and in many animals with present techniques an impossible one, but still not without a certain appeal. The principles which would be revealed, if such a conceptualization were adequate, are those allowing patterns of receptor stimulation to be classed as equivalent even though they are in detail different.

Couched within these terms, a principal problem for the

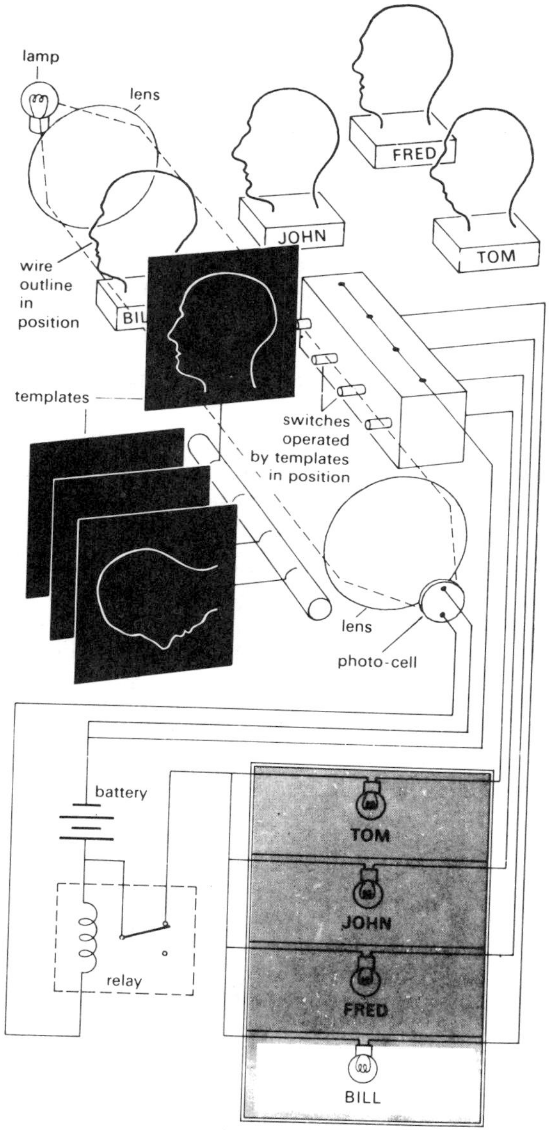

Figure 4.2 Illustration of the principle of template matching: when a given wire outline is arranged correctly a matching template can be selected to 'recognise' (classify) the pattern and produce a particular response (from Oatley, 1972).

nervous system is just how this classification of patterns of excitation on the organism's receptor surface and on subsequent interneurone networks occurs so that linkage of the outputs of classifiers can be made to particular responses. The nature of such a scheme in simple form is as shown in fig. 4.2 in which outline figures are classified according to whether they fit particular templates, and are thus enabled to operate particular responses. Template matching devices can be freed of the restriction of requiring a standardized input to the template by various preliminary operations, e.g. systematic sweeping of the image across the template would allow a response invariant of the position of the stimulus pattern, sweeping with a zoom lens would allow independence of size and so on. In neurophysiological examples the complex cells of Hubel and Weisel (1962) might be thought of as performing the equivalent of this first operation, and achieving a classification for any of a series of positions of a correctly oriented stimulus in the receptive field. They may do so be being responsive to all or any of the simple cells detecting stimuli in particular positions within the field.

A recent interest of neurophysiologists has been in the neurones which separate 'sustained' from 'transient' information into different channels in the visual system (e.g. Ikeda and Wright, 1974); the former being proposed as concerned with form vision and the latter with movement and change. Typically single units seem to respond best to some aspect of the stimulus pattern, and in so doing both separate information, and classify as equivalent many patterns which differ in detail, simply on the basis of a common denominator. The classification of visual movement by many animals independently of what is moving obeys these rules, and in some species that stimulus pattern alone may evoke responses of turning towards the place where movement occurred by means of arrangements for controlling the eye muscles (Oyster, 1968).

There have been variations on this 'stimulus classification' formulation of the functions of neuronal networks, namely that the networks act as filters, rejecting irrelevant aspects of the stimulus pattern (e.g. Barlow, 1961) or as transforming operations (e.g. Ratliff, 1965; Bekesy, 1967; Pollen and Taylor, 1974). In the first of these the notion is very much as I have already described: namely that by responding to some 'common denominator' of the image array, e.g. movement, a neurone or neurone network responds only to that aspect, rejecting irrelevant features, e.g. about brightness.

The second idea of neuronal networks as transform operators is like the idea that in order to make a template matching operation work, the raw pattern must be operated upon in some uniform way (e.g. by systematically changing size or position) so that a putative 'match' can be sought. Along these lines the operation of lateral inhibition can be seen as a transform which takes a matrix of points of varying brightness, and delivers an array of points in which the brightness gradient function (i.e. edges and lines in the picture) is displayed. An input array is operated on in some way (e.g. spatial differentiation, or convolution with a weighting function representing receptive field characteristics). The result is to deliver an array in terms not of the original brightness points, but in terms of changes (gradients) of brightness. Again as in the filtering notion, the idea is that this transformed array has characteristics in which the particularities of the raw stimulus array have been diminished or eliminated, and the hopefully significant generalities are transmitted. Operations of this kind probably are important in vision (see chapters 7 and 8), but if filtering and transforming operations are seen as ancillary to a classification scheme, we are not necessarily much further forward. We still have exactly the notion that neuronal networks exist to detect 'stimuli' in the receptor array.

Part of the interest of the classificatory arrangement (with or without notions of filtering and transforming) that has been developed for single neurone response is that it fits so readily into the ethologists' description of the releasing stimulus or sign stimulus (e.g. Tinbergen, 1951). As mentioned in the previous chapter, such a stimulus is that aspect of an event of biological importance to a particular animal to which it is sensitive, and by which the response is controlled. Perhaps the most striking example of this is in the tick, described by von Uexküll (1934). In the tick's world just three events are important: each is detected in terms of the presence of a single aspect of the situation, and each stimulus to which the tick is sensitive triggers a particular response. Thus when butyric acid is detected in the air, the tick releases its grasp on the branch from which it was hanging. It happens that butyric acid is a chemical secreted by the skin of mammals, and by letting go the branch when it detects this chemical it stands a good chance of landing on the back of a suitable host passing beneath it. Just as the zoologist classifies mammals by whether they suckle their young or have fur, the tick classifies them by whether or not they produce butyric acid. But unlike the zoologist, the tick when it is in the tree is quite insensitive to any other aspect of mammals. The tick is also equipped to detect mechanical stimulation from its host's hair. This stimulus causes the response of crawling about. Lastly it detects heat, and this causes it to bore into the host's skin. Thus events relevant to the life of the tick might plausibly be detected simply by receptors sensitive to butyric acid, mechanical stimulation, and warmth. What neurophysiology in the last twenty years has achieved is the rather strong evidence that not just chemical, mechanical or thermal stimuli can be sorted into independent categories constituted by separate neural pathways, but so too can much more complex patterns of receptor stimulation. A recent result of this kind is that of Updyke (1974) who found neurones in the superior colliculus of monkeys which responded to 'real' objects, such as the experimenter, but not to the usual stimuli or pictures projected onto the screen in front of the animal in the 'ordinary way'. Perhaps by connecting the right classifying cells or arrays of such cells to appropriate response-producing networks, behaviour can be produced.

It has been suggested as a result of ethological investigations that even quite complex behaviour can be produced in this kind of way. For instance, Lorenz (1969) cites the example of a complex genetically specified mechanism of this kind in a tame, young, hand-reared raven, which had never attacked, or seen an attack on, living prey. When it was released among a flock of jackdaws it made a determined dash at one to kill it with a well aimed blow at the back of its skull. Furthermore in the normal course of events a raven would stand no chance of catching a healthy and alert jackdaw. Evidently the raven singles out a jackdaw which is not so fit as the others, and thus offers the promise of a successful attack. The raven possesses a mechanism for releasing the behaviour of prey catching and killing in response to irregularities in the prey's locomotor activity. 'A slight stumbling, an irregularity of wing beat, or the like elicits a predatory attack with the mechanical predictability of a reflex, as trainers of big carnivores have learned to their cost.'

This kind of behaviour has been observed in wolves (Mech, 1971). Evidently wolves have no chance of catching a swift running caribou, so much so that a group of caribou will graze apparently peacefully and unconcerned in the presence of wolves. Yet the wolves will single out prospective prey, presumably again by detecting some sign of weakness or unhealthiness in a single animal, and launch an attack with may be successful. The question is this: some aspect of the unfit prey seems to trigger an attack in a reflex fashion, but is the event of interest (that a particular animal is unfit) understood by the predator? Or alternatively is recognition done on the cheap, by some simple aspect of the situtation being detected (as the tick detects butyric acid)? More generally the question is whether this type of reflex account will serve for all behaviour, and the answer on the stimulus side depends on whether in all cases, aspects of the environment with respect to which behaviour is organized can be classified as particular patterns of excitation of the receptor surface. In other words, is all perception equivalent to the classification of stimuli?

Over the last twenty years sensory neurophysiology has made a strong bid to resolve this problem about how far the idea of a stimulus, as a receptor excitation or the classification of patterns of receptor excitation, is a useful or a complete one in describing an animal's acquisition of information about the world. The following questions can be answered with some confidence. As to whether classificatory judgments are of importance in the life of animals, the ethological evidence is quite convincing. Many behaviour patterns do seem to be released on reception of signals denoting the presence of some characteristic and invariant aspect of environmental stimulation. Moreover, in many of the cases studied in detail, the stimulus is some very simple aspect of the situation, which is particularly prominent, and particularly discriminable. In some of these cases, the animal is easily fooled by artificial stimuli which exhibit this aspect of the stimulus.

Extending the idea further in the familiar psychological experiments of discrimination between various shapes and patterns it is clear that animals of most kinds can recognize (i.e. classify) stimuli, and that in many of the reported experiments the basis for the classification has been not the particular retinal image, but some aspect or dimension or feature of the stimulus patterns such as colour or orientation of lines.

It has been found, furthermore, that neural networks are capable of classifying such stimulus aspects as 'red' or 'horizontal' and even more complex aspects, such as 'real three dimensional objects' and in many cases such classifications are relatively independent of the precise conditions of luminance, retinal positon and size.

It seems, therefore, as if the findings of ethology and neurophysiology might be on the way to vindication of Descartes' rather bold suggestion that when those who fall from a height thrust out their hands to protect their heads, they do so not because of the appreciation of danger as such, but because some aspect of the dangerous situation, e.g. perhaps the sudden expansion of visual texture, acts as a stimulus. Some feature of the receptor pattern is classified by neuronal networks and selects the appropriate response. It certainly seems as if this is the correct analysis for the behaviour of the tick described by von Uexküll; it seems likely for the Roeder's (1966) moths avoiding bats on the basis of detecting their predators' echo locating squeaks, plausible for many of the 'released' behaviour patterns of vertebrates, and perhaps by extending the analysis to include learning it might be extended to include most behaviour. Was Descartes being too timid when he left in his scheme the unscientific notion of the soul? With a more clear sighted rationalism, we can see that our higher processes are learned, personally or culturally, so that we need not necessarily postulate some mysterious extra process, simply we must discover how new connections between stimulus and response are formed adaptively by the individual when he or she learns.

Or so the argument goes.

The problem of learning

The problem of the mechanism of learning has come to be thought of as one of the key issues in understanding neurophysiology and psychology. The reasons for this seem to be that by common consent learning is one of the things that people do extremely well and its value is seen in the way our education system seems to reward those individuals who do it best. Amongst other things, lower animals are lower in that it is supposed that they have lesser abilities to learn, less adaptability, less intelligence. It is superior learning ability perhaps which separates humans from animals, intelligence from simple machines composed of innate reflexes.

Pavlov (1927) was quite clear as to the object of his investigations of conditioning. It was to understand the higher, i.e. learned nervous processes. Tracing the theoretical derivation of his work from 'Descartes' idea of the nervous reflex ... a genuine scientific conception, since it implies necessity', he argued that the study of acquired reflexes was the business of physiology, and that there was nothing important to be learned from psychology, which had no claim to being an exact science. 'Conditioned reflexes', Pavlov argued, 'are phenomena of common and widespread occurrence: their establishment is an integral function in everyday life. We recognise them in ourselves and in other people under such names as "education", "habits", and "training"; and all of these are really nothing more than the results of an establishment of new nervous connections during the post natal existence of the organism. They are, in actual fact, links connecting definite extraneous stimuli with their definite responsive reactions.' Pavlov continued by saying that study of these reflexes would allow 'true physiological investigation probably of all the highest nervous activities of the cerebral hemispheres.'

Pavlov's complete identification of learning with higher nervous processes is both typical, and influential. It has been accompanied by the idea that there is a well formed question 'What is the nature of learning?' The assumption is that an answer to this question would tell us something important about how the brain works. This question phrased within the explicit or implicit structure of reflex theory can have only one interpretation 'What is the nature of the changes in connections between stimulus and response?' Or if one prefers a less neurological phrasing the logical content of which is exactly the same 'What is the nature of the laws relating stimulus to response under changes of environmental conditions?' We thus find physiologists searching for these connections and psychologists searching for these laws, both with the conviction that their discovery will throw a powerful light on the nature of learning and hence of higher nervous functions.

At the physiological level in the present climate of research it seems reasonable to suppose that the problem of changing interconnections during learning must focus on synapses, the switches in the pathways joining stimuli and responses. Clearly, therefore, any processes by which functional synaptic contact is formed, altered or discontinued are obvious candidates for physiological mechanisms of learning. Moreover, since synapses are mostly chemical, then it is to transmitter metabolism that one might look for such changes.

The basic logic of experiments on transmitter substances derives from standard neuropharmacological procedures developed for work on peripheral synapses. For the transmitter acetylcholine, for instance, there is within the synaptic cleft and on the post synaptic membrane an enzyme, acetyl cholinesterase, which inactivates the transmitter. This inactivation of acetylcholine diminishes both the amplitude and time constant of decay of post synaptic potentials. There are drugs which prevent the action of the cholinesterase enzymes (anticholinesterases), and these have the effect of increasing the amount of acetylcholine transmitter successfully crossing the synapse, and typically increasing the size of and prolonging post synaptic potentials.

Pharmacological manoeuvres of this kind applied in the context of various learning situations might, therefore, be expected to yield important conclusions about the physiological bases of learning. There are many typical experimental attempts.

One programme of research in this area of the relation of transmitters to environmental experience has been by Rosenzweig (e.g. 1970, 1972) and his colleagues Bennett and Diamond. Their basic finding is that rats raised from birth in enriched environments, i.e. ten or twelve rats to a large cage which is equipped with running wheels, ladders and other paraphernalia, acquire thicker cerebral cortices, and changes in the amount of cortical acetylcholinesterase, as compared with litter mates living alone in small rat cages with no objects to manipulate. The specific enzyme acetylcholinesterase, though it is in absolute terms increased in quantity in the rats with enriched early experience, is decreased in comparison with their total mass of cortex. Non-specific cholinesterase activity mainly attributable to giant cells, on the other hand, is increased both absolutely and relatively. The enriched early environment has also been found to assist rats in improving on a series of reversals of a discrimination task.

Somewhat more specifically, Kerkut, Oliver, Rick and Walker (1970) have made biochemical studies of Horridge's

(1965) phenomenon of leg raising by a headless cockroach in which only a single thoracic ganglion controls the response to electric shock. Three groups of preparations were used: experimental animals were given shocks to the leg at the rate of 1 per second, all the time that the leg dipped into a saline solution. Yoked control animals were given exactly the same number of shocks at the same instant as the experimentals, but the shocks were not contingent upon leg position of the control animals. Resting animals received no shocks. The experimental preparation learned to keep its leg out of the saline in about 35 minutes; but the other animals did not. Kerkut *et al* found that anti-cholinesterase drugs, such as prostigmine, speeded learning, so that experimental animals reached criterion in about 15 instead of 35 minutes. Also, estimates of the amount of cholinesterase in the ganglion fell to about one third during the course of the normal 35 minutes learning period, gradually returning to normal over a period of three days. The three days exactly coincided with the period over which the cockroach ganglion effectively forgot the response. A second change during learning in which experimentals were different from controls or resting animals was in an increased amount of GABA, a supposedly inhibitory transmitter. If acetylcholine were an excitatory transmitter in this system, then the decrease in cholinesterase and increase in GABA would both be expected to have a facilitatory synaptic effect, which in this case would presumably operate somewhere in the pathway leading to motorneurones lifting the leg.

The same type of reasoning, though with some slightly more exotic postulates, has been employed by Deutsch (1971) in his search for a basic cholinergic mechanism underlying learning in rats. Deutsch argued that when the amount of acetylcholine released at a synapse is small, or the sensitivity of the post synaptic membrane is low, then the effect of moderate doses of anticholinesterase agents is to facilitate cholinergic transmission. On the other hand, if there is a lot of acetylcholine being released at a synapse or post synaptic sensitivity is high, anticholinesterases have the effect of increasing the amount of acetylcholine so much that it blocks the synapse completely. Thus anticholinesterase can be used with success to treat myaesthenia gravis, helping to strengthen the weak muscular contractions characteristic of the disease, which are thought to be due to diminished transmitter. The same dose of the drug in a normal person produces paralysis. If memory involves changes in acetylcholine released at a synapse or change in sensitivity of the post synaptic membrane, then cholinesterase given at a stage where synapses were transmitting weakly might be expected to facilitate performance, but giving it when a task was well learned and well remembered might block the synapse altogether.

Deutsch went on to demonstrate exactly this effect in discriminated avoidance tasks. Intracranial injections of the anticholinesterase drug di-iopropyl fluorophosphate (DFP) greatly facilitated correct performance on a poorly learned difficult discrimination, between dim light and darkness, but on an easy discrimination between a bright light and darkness that had been well learned in the same number of trials, the anticholinesterase had a large depressive effect on performance. In another experiment DFP injected three weeks after training had a facilitatory effect on performance of the partly forgotten task, but when injected only seven days after the task was learned, it blocked performance.

Extinction, as is clear from other evidence (such as the phenomenon of spontaneous recovery), is not to be explained by a weakening of synaptic connectivity of the same synapse that subserved acquisition. Deutsch indicated that it is subserved by another set of cholinergic synapses. He concludes that discrimination learning probably involves an increase in sensitivity of post synaptic membranes in cholinergic synapses (but an increase in the amount of learning does not recruit more synapses). Following acquisition, the post synaptic membranes continue to become more sensitive for a few days and then sensitivity declines; this decline being the process underlying forgetting. An initial decrease in responsiveness to cholinesterase a few minutes after learning, might, Deutsch supposes, be due to a parallel set of synapses with fast decay subserving short term memory.

From experiments of this kind it seems quite possible to conclude that acetylcholine transmitter processes are involved in learning as defined by the kinds of experiments designed by psychologists.

Psychologists, of course, may take the view that they do not have much to say about the actual connections themselves but are exercised to understand the logical (rather than the physiological) dependency of response on stimulus. Skinner for instance is one such.

In *The Behaviour of Organisms* (1938) Skinner laid out a system of behavioural description which had as its principal terms stimulus, response, and reflex. Skinner defines stimulus as that part or aspect of the environment that affects behaviour, response as the correlated part of behaviour affected by the environment. Neither stimulus nor response 'may be defined as to its essential properties without the other.'

The observed relation between stimulus and response is termed the reflex. So defined, Skinner claims, the reflex is not a theory but a fact, and is indeed 'an analytical unit which makes an investigation of behaviour possible.' It is not the only unit, however; some responses are not elicited by any environmental stimuli; they are emitted spontaneously, and these responses Skinner calls operants. Although previously the term reflex was used to describe only respondent behaviour in which an environmental stimulus elicited a response, Skinner extended its use to include operant behaviour in which responses were emitted, without environmental provocation, but were then brought under the control of stimuli. Such stimuli are (a) reinforcing stimuli, the 'effects' which Thorndike (1911) described, in his 'law of effect' and which through learning alter the probability of responses which precede them, and (b) discriminative stimuli the occurrences of which are correlated with the appearance of reinforcement, and come through learning to 'set the occasion for a response.' Discriminative stimuli in this scheme though differing from eliciting stimuli correspond rather closely to conditioned stimuli in classical conditioning in that they both signal a biologically important event and through learning come to control the occurrence of responses.

Skinner is careful to state that he believes his scheme to be simply a description of behaviour and that his systemization is independent of neurology. Thus for instance the term 'reflex' should be taken merely as implying a relationship between stimulus and response not as asserting that the relationship is supported by any particular type of neural connection. Skinner's argument that psychology can be pursued independently of any reference to brain tissue is perfectly sound. Though it stands in sharp distinction to the attitude of Pavlov (1927) who claimed his conditioning experiments to be a means of investigating the physiology of the cerebral cortex.

By no means all those interested in animal learning follow

Skinner's analysis. Many regard it as important not just to define laws relating stimuli to responses under complicated schedules of reinforcement, but to work more directly towards establishing a theory of the logical structure of what goes on in the middle, between the stimulus and the response.

One of the most influential recent theories, for instance, that of Rescorla and Wagner (1972) is a quite formal mathematical theory for Pavlovian conditioning with two conditioned stimuli (usually a light and a tone). The equations predict the course of conditioning in terms of the strength of responses made to stimuli, including various odd effects that occur for instance when animals are conditioned in the presence of both stimuli, and are then tested with only one. Taking the form of a pair of equations the theory is quite unequivocal in its assumptions and predictions, and this is clearly an important property.

It needs to be pointed out, moreover, that some people working in the field of animal learning now rather energetically refute the idea that they are trying to understand stimulus-response connections. One rather sly form this takes is the current emphasis on classical conditioning as an experimental paradigm (as in Rescorla and Wagner's work). Here the response is taken as trivial, and used only as an index of the association between events (stimuli).

More radically, some of these theorists now cast their work into a different framework. For instance Rescorla (personal communication) has expressed agreement to the proposition that he was trying to create a competence model of the animal's perception of causality in the environment. Recently Mackintosh (1976) has written along the same lines, that in general the idea of looking for 'associative' processes in animal learning consists of discovering the animal's perceptions and conceptions of causality in the environment. One set of observations are, for instance, that the strength of conditioning depends upon how well an event predicts reinforcement in the environment as compared to other less good predictors (candidates for causing the reinforcement).

There are, of course, very many other psychological approaches to animal learning, both for Pavlovian and instrumental conditioning. Animal learning theory is, however, completely unanimous in one regard. All accounts take stimuli or stimulus dimensions as inputs, all produce some aspect of a response as (for instance, response strength, probability of a particular response) an output. So the task does seem to be seen as defining the logic of the production of responses from stimuli in learning tasks, the laws of association among stimuli, or between stimuli and responses.

Obviously there are variations: theories where reinforcement is emphasized, theories which suppose that the connection between stimulus and response is what is learned, theories which suppose that animals learn not the response of a particular movement, but the response of approaching a particular stimulus and so on. But no learning theory takes seriously the problem of having to interact with the real world, by, for instance, analysing an input from a retinal image or equivalent, or by wandering robot-like around the environment. It is assumed that stimuli are categorized, and that responses can be made, and that how these things occur is the concern in the quite different and separable problems of perception and motor control. Learning takes place in a compartment which accepts stimuli and emits responses. The job of learning theory is to define what goes on in that compartment, by designing experiments in which animals are confronted with what the experimenter defines as stimuli, in environments such as Skinner boxes and mazes designed to detect what the experimenter defines as the response of interest. The whole enterprise takes place implicitly or explicitly within the conceptual framework of learning being a change of response consequent on changes in the stimulus, in other words, within the theory of reflexes: stimuli, connections, and responses.

The quest for the understanding of learning is seen as important in animals and man, because it seems to epitomize 'higher' nervous or mental processes. Within the theory the quest has a well defined direction, whether it is conceived in the physiological or psychological terms. The direction cannot be other than trying to discover how responses relate or connect to stimuli.

Levels of function in the nervous system

One theme which was explicit in Descartes' account of nervous action, and which has been energetically developed subsequently is the idea of higher and lower aspects of behaviour, and their identification with different parts of the nervous system. In this account lower parts of the brain are supposed to be taken up with reflex machinery, while higher processes of mind act by influence on these basic mechanisms.

The main developer of this theme was the Victorian neurologist, Hughlings Jackson (two volumes of whose selected works were published in 1958). Jackson's writing was rambling, diffuse and repetitive, but it contained, nevertheless, some fundamental ideas which in one way or another have permeated the thinking of almost all later workers on the brain. He was much influenced by Spencer's (1899) evolutionary theory and considered higher regions of the brain (the midbrain and cortex) to be evolved from the lower regions such as the spinal cord. This evolution involved a change from highly organized and simple mechanisms to ones which were complex and as yet unorganized. These later products of evolution were unorganized in the sense that they were still in the process of becoming organized, by learning for example. In a human brain, therefore, the cortex was the highest level, while successively lower levels were more automatic, more organized and more simple.

Systems of movement were arranged hierarchically, so that whereas at the lowest level, organization was that of a single reflex involving for instance only an isolated part of the body or a single flexion movement, at the next higher level this same movement would be represented again but now co-ordinated with other movements and parts of the body. At the highest level of the cortex the body parts and movements would be represented again in (Jackson's word is re- re-represented) but now in total combination of all parts in terms of their 'most special and complex combinations'.

Each higher level thus exerted control over the lower one, but the higher levels were more fragile and thus more liable to be taken out of service either locally (by discrete lesions) or generally across a whole level by various neurological afflictions, and this removal of control by higher levels represented a process opposite to evolution, namely dissolution.

Jackson expresses the relationship between levels quite clearly in the following (politically rather questionable) metaphor.

> The higher nervous arrangements evolved out of the lower, keep down those lower, just as a government evolved out of a

> nation controls as well as directs that nation. If this be the process of evolution then the reverse process of dissolution is not only a 'taking off' of the higher, but is at the very same time 'letting go' of the lower. If the governing body of this nation were destroyed suddenly we should have two causes for lamentation: (1) the loss of services of eminent men; and (2) the anarchy of the now uncontrolled people.

In drunkenness, argued Jackson, we see just this general release from higher control. In certain kinds of neurological injury, moreover, Jackson claims that we might find a person with a speech defect. His only speech is to say 'yes' and 'no'. In answer to a question 'Is your name Jones?', he says 'No', a lower, more automatic response, but ask him 'Please say no', a more voluntary response, and he cannot. Removal of all but the lowest level in Jacksonian terms is coma, with only such functions as respiration and the heartbeat still operating.

Jackson's illustrations of his doctrine are extraordinarily extensive, and like some of the above not always totally convincing. But his marshalling of what had been an incoherent mass of neurological symptoms under such principles as that pathological behaviour arises as a result of release from higher control of some mechanism already present was remarkable.

Jackson himself was not an experimenter, and some of the ideas he espoused, such as that the seat of the higher functions of volition and perception was in the cortex, had already been expounded by the influential French physiologist, Flourens (1824), on the basis of experimental brain transections. Subsequent experiments have revealed that the removal of the upper parts of the brain, or transection of the brain to leave only the spinal cord communicating with the muscles, very markedly simplify an animal's behavioural repertoire. As Sherrington (1906) observed, transection of the brain to leave only the spinal cord intact reduces the animal to a reflex automaton of exactly the kind that Descartes had postulated. The animal with only its spinal cord responds only when stimulated, and is capable of no self-initiated behaviour. So, for instance, Bard (1940) has shown that a female cat with spinal cord severed from its brain will make reflex treading movements, crouch, deflect its tail and make other movements associated with copulation when its vagina is stimulated with a glass rod. Without stimulation the cat is passive and motionless. A cat with more of the nervous system including the hypothalamus intact and connected to the spinal cord, but with the cortex disconnected, is under some 'higher' control, and makes these reflex actions on genital stimulation, only when female sex hormones are circulating in the blood. (The spinal cat is uninfluenced by hormones.) Such an animal, without a cortex, when in heat or when supplied artificially with hormones will not seek out sexual contact, or approach distant male animals as does the cat with the brain entirely intact. The results of transecting the brain at different levels thus correspond well with Hughlings Jackson's idea of behaviour being constrained to different levels of complexity.

Teitelbaum (1967), one recent expositor of the theory of levels and of simplification of behaviour by lesions, interprets these results as indicating that in the spinal cord are organized the simple automatic reflexes in which neuronal chains connect stimulus to response. Higher levels of the brain (up to and including the hypothalamus) modulate the activity of these reflex paths, and integrate reflexes together so that the rather isolated movements become joined into complete series of actions. They, furthermore, place reflex responsivity under control intrinsic to the organism. Thus hormones modulate sexual receptivity, deficits of water initiate drinking behaviour and so on. The organism with this level of function is said to behave at the level of instinct, with relevant mechanisms including those of hormonal sensitivity localized primarily in the middle level of the diencephalon. Voluntary behaviour, according to Teitelbaum, and as both Jackson and Flourens had supposed, is associated with the cerebral hemispheres. Flourens concluded, for instance, that perception, memory, judgment and volition all reside here. The more modern Teitelbaum rephrases this by claiming that the hemispheres are the area required for operant conditioning. Taking the idea somewhat further, a number of authors, e.g. Luria (1970), have claimed that the frontal part of the brain is the highest level of all, responsible for formation of intentions and programmes of behaviour.

Thus the progression from lower to higher parts of the brain is associated with the progression from lower to higher aspects of behaviour. The analysis suggests several corollaries.

In ontogenetic development, for instance, the reflexes of the newborn baby give way to instinctive patterns, and then to volition and to progressively more sophisticated behaviour as progressively higher parts of the nervous system become active. Thus, Teitelbaum (1967) traces the establishment of these successive levels of control in human infants. At first the baby behaves only reflexly, with approach reflexes such as moving her mouth towards something touching her on the cheek and sucking it, with withdrawal reflexes from painful stimuli, and various postural reflexes. As she grows up involuntary reflex and instinctive patterns can not be elicited by stimuli which would previously elicit them. By this time the basic reflex components of behaviour are still present but have come under the control of higher, voluntary mechanisms.

In the course of phylogenetic development too it is argued that there is a progression towards more complex behaviour. Quite explicit in Hughlings Jackson's doctrine of levels is the notion of higher levels being more highly evolved. It, therefore, comes as no surprise to find the ideas in the literature that phylogenetic evolution of the brain involves the acquisition of successively higher levels in the nervous system, and that this is responsible for successively more complex and sophisticated behaviour.

Sometimes, the dominant idea in trying to understand the relation between the nervous system and man's most prized 'higher' functions, is that mere bulk of brain is the important variable: more being better, in that it allows of greater complexity of nervous tissue to explain complexity of behaviour. Lashley's (e.g. 1929) idea of mass action (the idea that total mass of cortex independently of its specific location is the determinant of abilities like maze learning, and hence supposedly general properties such as intelligence) is clearly an example of this.

Stepping further out on a limb than Lashley was prepared to go we can even find attributions of consciousness to brains once they have reached a sufficient size, and hence sufficient complexity. Let's say indeed that this point is reached when a brain of about the size of man's evolves. A version of this argument, for instance, is put by Rose in his book of 1973 in a chapter entitled 'The evolution of brains and consciousness'. Consciousness, he declares, is a function of the number of cells in the brain perhaps of uncommitted neurones of the association cortex, and of the number of their connections with each other. As one ascends the phylogenetic scale from animals with only a few neurones to the final summit, man, there is an increase in the plastic capacity of behaviour, and an increase in brain to body weight ratio. This latter signifies an increasing value of the function of total neurones and their connectivity. This function Rose claims is of a type such that there is a significant quantitative break with the emergence of man. Once sufficient complexity is achieved, consciousness suddenly appears.

As these ideas of increasing complexity of brain and behaviour become more specific they typically focus on the evolution of the vertebrate brain. Here successive stages in the course of phylogenerate development do not just appear as producing brains that tip weighing scales at successively higher values, but as structural additions to identifiable parts of the nervous system, whose properties and functions we might, therefore, be able to investigate.

The phylogenetic development of the vertebrates is thought to have been from fish to amphibia to reptiles, with birds and mammals as independent branches from the reptile stem. The neurological accompaniments of this phylogenetic progression up the stem and mammalian branch of this tree may be characterized as an increase in size of the forebrain, and in particular, the addition and enlargement of the cerebral cortex (Jerison, 1973).

In so far as the phylogenetic development can be reflected by modern species, this progression is deduced from the observation that fish have no cortex; and amphibia and reptiles have only a very tiny cortex. (In birds the cortex is small in comparison with the rest of the brain but there has been a substantial increase in the size of the midbrain.)

In mammals the cerebral cortex becomes the most noticeable structure in the brain, becoming more pronounced in the progression from marsupials via intermediate forms such as rodents to primates. The progression culminates in man who not only has a very large brain in absolute terms, with a larger number of nerve cells and interconnections than other forms, but with the enlargement mainly in the cerebral cortex.

One attack on this problem which illustrates well the preoccupation with higher levels of the brain being added in evolution and being concerned with supposedly higher aspects of behaviour has been undertaken by Bitterman (e.g. 1965).

He enquired whether corticalization provides a basis for a progressive increase in intelligence, by training a variety of animals (fish, turtle, pigeon, rat and monkey) on simultaneous discrimination tasks which required either a position habit (left versus right) or a visual discrimination (e.g. black versus white) for solution. In one kind of test with this task, he investigated how well these animals learned successive reversals.

For instance, on the spatial task if the animal had been rewarded for choosing the left side until it reached a criterion of correct performance over a number of trials, the reward was then reversed, i.e. switched to the right side until the criterion of correct performance was again reached. Then the reward was switched back to the left side, and so forth. Monkeys, rats and pigeons improved their speed of learning with successive reversals with both visual and spatial tasks. Fish, however, did not: they took exactly as long to learn the twentieth reversal as they did to learn the task originally. Turtles were intermediate. They improved on successive spatial reversals, but not on reversals of the visual task.

In another variation of the discrimination task Bitterman rewarded one side (or one visual stimulus) for instance 70% of the time, while the other was rewarded 30% of the time on a pseudo-random schedule. The 'intelligent' thing to do in such a task is to choose always the stimulus that is rewarded 70% of the time. This Bitterman calls maximizing; monkeys, rats and birds did this. Fish, on the other hand, distributed their responses roughly in the proportion that the rewards were distributed, i.e. they responded 70% to the stimulus rewarded 70% of the time and 30% to the stimulus rewarded 30% of the time. Performing in this way, which was called matching, resulted in their collecting only 58% (70% of 70% plus 30% of 30%) of the possible rewards, as opposed to 70% that they could have collected by maximizing. Turtles again were intermediate, and matched on the visual task, but maximized on the spatial one.

What now happens if a rat's brain is reduced to the level of a lower animal? Gonzalez, Roberts and Bitterman (1964) have performed this experiment by removing the greater part of the rats' cortices in infancy, and testing them on reversals and probability learning in adulthood. They found that these decorticate rats behaved rather like turtles (which also have only a small piece of cortex) failing to improve on successive reversals of a visual task, but improving quite normally on spatial reversals, and maximizing on a left-right discrimination, but matching on a black-white task.

A more improbable piece of surgery has been to increase the intellectual resources of a fish, by grafting on an extra piece of brain. Bresler and Bitterman (1969) found that by transplanting material into the prospective tectal region of embryo mouth-breeding fish they were able in some individuals to increase the size of the tectal area of the brain in the adult. The survival rate for this operation was low, but of four fish who survived and had increased brain size, two learned a visual task and reversals with many fewer errors than normal fish or than transplanted fish, which turned out to have histologically normal brains. Two fish with increased brainpower improved on successive reversals; a performance not characteristic of fish at all, but associated with the learning of 'higher animals'.

There are formidable difficulties in trying to order behavioural abilities in an evolutionary sequence of behaviour, to correlate these with an evolutionary progression of intelligence, and to correlate both these with a sequence of brain morphology. Some of these difficulties, as pointed out by Hodos (1970), spring from the fact that the course of vertebrate evolution is not fully understood. But more problems arise in behavioural analysis because there is effectively no behavioural equivalent of the fossil record. There are some behavioural fossils: evidence of the use of fire, flint tools, holes in the heads of presumably hunted animals that seem to have been made by blunt instruments, and so on. But these are all confined to anthropoids and are comparatively recent.

A problem of working with existing, that is to say, modern, animals is that each of these has had exactly as long a history of evolution as man has, and each species is well adapted to its environment. If it were not, it would not be here. Thus if a fish, or a turtle, a rat, or whatever, shows some aspect of behaviour, or learns in a particular way, this is just as likely to represent an adaptation to the exigencies of that animal's ecological niche, as evidence for possession or otherwise of any general intelligence. These and many other objections to Bitterman's experiments have been made. I do not wish to discuss their validity here, but to point out that Bitterman's experiments, whether or not they are (as he claims) the best that can be done in impossible circumstances, represent the outcome of a very pervasive theory in brain research: the idea of higher accretions of the brain making for higher abilities. Bitterman's use of surgery to produce regression to more primitive forms and advance to more complex ones, thus directly continues the tradition of Hughlings Jackson.

The notion of levels of function permeates brain research in other ways too. Thus, for instance, Vanderwolf (1971) distinguishes between lower involuntary movements such as shivering, chewing, grooming, which are automatically connected to particular (instinctive) mechanisms. Voluntary behaviour patterns such as walking originate in the cortex and are accompanied by different patterns of electrical activity in various parts of the brain. These movements are voluntary in that any one can be temporarily brought into the service of any motivational state.

The division between the entirely automatic and the higher voluntary is not absolute though. Miller (e.g. 1971) and his associates in a series of experiments have shown that responses of the autonomic nervous system, long considered (at least in the western world) to be beyond voluntary control can be modified by instrumental learning techniques. Thus heart rate, blood flow through peripheral vessels, the rate of urine production have all been reported to be capable of modification in anaesthetized animals by rewarding changes of these parameters with intracranial electrical stimulation. These phenomena, though they have declined in impressiveness since first reported, and though testifying to the flexibility of behaviour, do not contradict the notion that in general the autonomic nervous system is usually automatic. It can and does in the ordinary way carry on its business without voluntary interference. However, Miller's findings were surprising precisely because they seemed to contradict this very widely held view.

As described in the previous section the idea of higher functions has often been taken as synonymous with learning ability. Thus Pavlov announced that his discovery of conditioning put within reach the objective study of all higher nervous functions. Subsequently many demonstrations of the confinement of the apparently more complex kinds of learning ability to the cortex have been given. Perhaps the best known are the split-brain demonstrations of Sperry (e.g. 1967, 1974) and his colleagues. The surgical operation to split the brain involves severing the corpus callosum and other tracts connecting the left and right halves of the cortex. Split-brain cats, monkeys, and even people (who have had this operation to relieve certain kinds of epilepsy) seem in many respects to be entirely normal. But if stimuli are presented on only one side of the body their neurophysiological consequences reach only one side of the cortex, and anything learned on one side, e.g. a visual discrimination associating reward with a triangle but not a square, stays on that side and is not available to the other. Thus if the stimuli are shown to the side that did not learn the discrimination, no knowledge of their significance exists, and indeed an entirely contradictory discrimination (e.g. that reward is associated with the square) can be taught to that side. The learning process and the information stored must, therefore, be cortical, it is claimed, for if it were subcortical, access to it in the split brain preparation would be equally easy from either side.

Certain forms of learning e.g. habituation (Spencer, Thompson and Nielson, 1966) can occur at the low level of the isolated spinal cord. Classical conditioning on the other hand, needs higher levels, but can occur in decorticated animals (e.g. Girden *et al*, 1930). The doctrine of levels thus seems to confirm (though by a rather circular argument) suspicions that habituation and classical conditioning have the status of lower forms of learning. It is instrumental learning, which seems to require that at least some cortex be present, and is by the same token, a higher form of learning.

Further research on the split brain has extended the notion of levels with the suggestion that though at birth left and right hemispheres are equal in potentialities, by some kind of struggle one, usually the left, comes to dominate the other and controls the most skilled movements, of the preferred hand, as well as being responsible for speech, which is thought of as being a higher activity. In a rare individual genetically lacking a corpus callosum, speech has been found represented on both sides. Thus, one function of this huge tract of fibres, Sperry argues, is to allow one hemisphere to establish so called 'dominance' over the other. The hemispheres are arranged side by side, and although some people e.g. Milner (1974) now argue for specialization rather than dominance in the analysis of these phenomena; in right-handed people the left hemisphere still seems to be thought of as representing a higher Jacksonian level than the right.

Another elaboration of doctrine of levels was provided by work on the reticular system. Though it is itself at a relatively 'low' level in the brain, the reticular system is not only influenced by superior levels, but can influence all levels above itself by alerting them. Had Hughlings Jackson had to comment on the role of this structure he might have likened it to the force of public opinion, which supposedly can keep a government on its toes, and make it acutely aware of some issue, but without making it clear what the proper course of action is.

One problem with the separation of the brain by surgical transections and ablations into a series of levels is that some of the conclusions that follow from these operations could scarcely be otherwise. It would be surprising indeed if behaviour became more complex, more ingenious or more insightful when large pieces of the organ that seems to be responsible for generating behaviour were removed. What is surprising and unlike our experience of most physical mechanisms is that so much brain can be removed and organized adaptive behaviour can still occur. The removal of some lower parts of the brain, e.g. the medulla, of course, results in no behaviour at all, complex or otherwise. But a removal of a part which does not result in death must if it has any effect, reduce the complexity of behaviour. Thus the discovery that 'higher' levels of the nervous system can be removed with greater impunity than 'lower', therefore, automatically produces a tendency to attribute elaborative (rather than basic) functions to these higher parts, and the doctrine of levels is in many ways a description of the behavioural consequences of these manipulations, couched in neurological terms.

The theory of levels in the nervous system has a very direct relationship with Descartes' theory of the reflex. This relationship can take one of three forms. A 'levels' theory follows Descartes exactly, simply elaborating the number of levels beyond the two (reflex and reasoning mind in the pineal) described by Descartes. This clearly is the version followed by Hughlings Jackson, and also that followed by people who talk about higher functions such as intelligence, consciousness or whatever, asserting that they have some embodiment in the higher parts of the brain, but without having anything much to say about their mechanism.

A second form the relationship of levels to reflex theory takes is that chosen by Pavlov, namely the assertion that reflexes are all that exist in the brain. In this case the notion 'higher', which is used freely by Pavlov simply comes to mean reflexes which are conditioned as opposed to reflexes which are innate: higher means learned. Descartes described the pineal as 'inclining successively to different sides ... until [the animal spirits] come upon that part where the traces are left of the thing which it [the mind] wishes to remember', in an attempt to say something about the relation of the higher level to the lower. Learned traces, he said, are 'nothing else than ... the pores of the brain through which the spirits have already taken their course on presentation of the object, and have thereby acquired a greater facility than the rest to be opened again'. Whereas Descartes was reticent about what moved the pineal, Pavlov simply identifies all higher mental processes with the formation of new pathways, thus removing the mystery from the domain of the pineal. The mind need not will to remember: the properties of conditioned pathways themselves constitute the will. A separate mind is unnecessary.

The third form which 'levels' and reflexes are related is that espoused by at least some hard-headed experimentalists. Though there may be elaborations, the basic pattern is clear. At the lowest level are simple reflexes. Stimuli are detected, come in along specific sensory pathways, and are connected by switches to appropriate response pathways. Higher levels mean one of two things, either (a) somewhat longer reflex pathways with more synapses between stimulus and response or (b) longer pathways still, which take off from and then reconnect with the lower reflex pathways. What is clear is that with higher levels meaning either multiplication of synapses, or modulation of lower reflex pathways, there is still only one mechanism that will fulfil the elementary criterion of being able to produce some behaviour: the stimulus-response reflex connection. Just as in the original Descartes model, this is the only mechanism producing behaviour, all any higher processes do in addition is to modify the connective pathways.

Higher levels may be said to inhibit or facilitate, modulate, co-ordinate, or integrate lower mechanisms. Some characteristics of higher level mechanisms can even be described (e.g. hormonal sensitivity), although as often as not the term 'higher processes' actually means processes whose nature is not well understood. Whatever their nature though, their operation must within the reflex theory necessarily be limited to tuning, increasing, or decreasing the conductivity of reflex pathways.

The mechanism of the reflex, as Descartes showed with his mechanical analogies, is unquestionably capable of producing some behaviour. The question remains: whether all behaviour can be composed from reflexes, or stimulus response connections. Some authors, for example Sherrington (1906) have implied that it can. 'The unit reaction in nervous integration is the reflex' he wrote. Rather in the same way as the basic anatomical unit is the neurone the basic behavioural unit is composed of the reflex arc, comprising receptor, conducting path, and effector. Arranged in the spinal cord, and in various parts of the hind-brain (the parts of the brain immediately forward of or above the cord) are the connections comprising these reflex arcs, the repertoire of behavioural component parts from which sequences of behaviour must be assembled.

In many ways Hughlings Jackson's ideas about levels are as good as those of anyone who has written subsequently. He ascribed to the brain the task operating with complex schemata of action; he supposed that the brain thought in terms of actions, not muscular movements. This emphasis on the problems of organization is itself a worthwhile elaboration of the reflex idea. He even introduced some new metaphors, such as the one about government and the 'lower orders', which help us think about these issues. But we still need to think about the brain with a richer set of metaphors and analogies. Although because of our experience of living in society we have quite good intuitions about Hughlings Jackson's metaphors, social metaphors are not enough. An analogy of this kind gives us a feeling for what might happen in the brain, but because we do not actually understand the workings of society we can not use it as productively as we might wish, to explain how the brain works.

Descartes' analogy has an easily understood mechanism. If the preceding arguments are correct, it is indeed the main concept of a mechanism capable of producing behaviour which underlies a great deal of research in this field.

In summary then, the doctrine of levels, like Descartes attribution of the mind to the pineal, can be seen as some sort of statement that reflexes are not enough. But we have an inadequate supply of analogies or metaphors that are any better. And since scientists like to talk about mechanism, rather than something more vague, it is still the reflex mechanism with dominates our thinking and understanding.

IMPLICATIONS AND INADEQUACIES OF THE THEORY

In the previous three sections I hope I have shown some ways in wich reflex theory pervades our understanding of the brain. I have not attempted comprehensive reviews of the literature, and I do not claim that the examples of research that I have chosen represent the only kinds of thinking that occur in the fields I have chosen. Rather I would claim that these examples are representative of the kinds of ways in which reflex theory, either explicitly or implicitly espoused tends to direct and constrain hypotheses and experiments. Sometimes one sees the theoretical banner waved boldly as for instance in the introduction to a section of a recent compendium of neurobiological knowledge, stating 'Much study of animal and human behaviour has yielded the following equation to which virtually everyone now adheres: Stimulus→Response'. The arrow 'sums up diagrammatically the laws of the brain by which the stimulus becomes connected with a response.' Sometimes the theory is less explicit. But the names to conjure with in understanding behaviour have for a long time been, and still are at least to an extent: stimulus, response, and the means whereby they are related.

Lashley spent much of his life trying experimentally to refute reflex theory. In his work on perception he was at pains to stress the equivalence of stimuli, the fact that a pattern was recognized as such independently of its size, or its precise location. In order to demonstrate this kind of phenomenon, Lashley (e.g. 1938) used the transfer test. A rat is trained with two stimuli, A and B, so that it is rewarded for jumping towards A but not rewarded for approaching B. After reaching a criterion of success in this performance, the animal is shown new stimuli, and the experimenter determines to what extent the animal treats new (test) stimuli like the original training stimuli. For instance, in one of his (1938) experiments rats were trained to approach the larger of two circular patches. After reaching criterion they were tested with a pair of circular patches consisting of the smaller training shape, and a yet smaller one. The rats still approached the larger of the test pair, but this was the original smaller negative stimulus, the actual one that during training the rats has learned to avoid.

In variations of this paradigm, Lashley trained rats to choose between, e.g. a solid vertical and a solid horizontal stripe, and then found that the discrimination held up with outline stripes, or dotted ones, or sets of thinner horizontal and vertical stripes. The conclusion is that if the rat treats a test stimulus in the same way as a physically different training stimulus, he is not responding to the particular retinal image, but to some more abstract quality that test and training stimulus have in common, for instance in these last two examples, relative size and orientation respectively.

As discussed in the section on 'The search for the adequate stimulus' one of the achievements of Hubel and Wiesel's (1962) work was the demonstration that neurones of the kind they called complex cells behaved in a way that seemed to acount for this latter (horizontal versus vertical) discrimination. These neurones responded selectively to particular orientations, somewhat independently of exact retinal position and of the precise form of the stimulus, provided it exhibited some orientation feature. From this kind of discovery it seemed possible that on looking further into the nervous system neurones with progressively more abstract classification properties would be found.

It is perhaps less clear how such pattern classification neurones could support a discrimination of relative size. As Lashley pointed out, animals and men respond to relational rather than absolute properties. It was on this kind of evidence that Lashley stated that despite the observation that 'nerve impulses are transmitted over definite restricted paths ... all behaviour seems to be determined by ... the form or relations or properties of excitation within general fields of activity. It is the pattern not the element that counts.'

A more modern demonstration of the fact that recognition does not depend simply on the particular retinal stimulation comes from Shepard and Metzler (1971). They showed some pairs of line drawings depicting fairly complex three-dimensional objects (see fig. 4.3). In one type of pair the patterns were the same. One was simply a rotation of the other, as if, say, the left hand one had been cut out and turned clockwise through a given number of degrees. In the second type the object depicted was the same in both pictures, but the

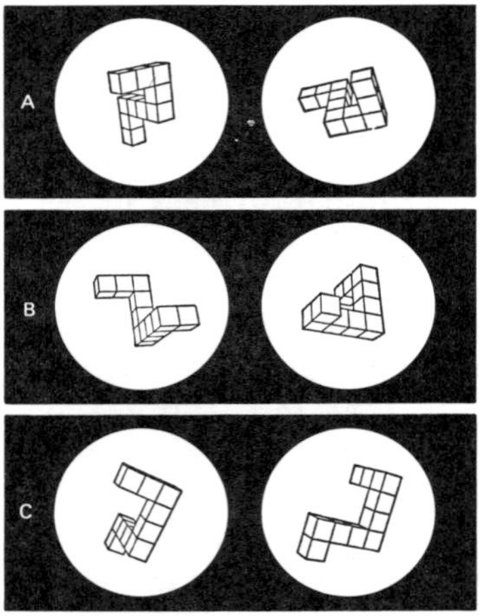

Figure 4.3 Pairs of objects shown by Shepard and Metzler:(a) the same objects with the right hand picture rotated; (b) the same objects but one rotated in depth with respect to the other; (c) the objects are different, they are mirror images. (From Shepard and Metzler, 1971).

two pictures were of the same object in different rotations in depth, i.e. round a vertical axis. Here the actual pictures were very different, one picture could not be cut out to superimpose upon the other. In the third type of pair the objects depicted were actually different.

Subjects were asked to say 'same' or 'different' on presentation of each of a mixed series of such pairs. They made few errors and furthermore were just as fast when members of the pair were versions rotated in-depth, as when they were rotations of the picture. In other words, despite the fact that when viewed from a single position, an object rotated about an axis, say, at right angles to the line of view presents a much changed retinal pattern, with parts seen from one view being invisible from another and with changed angles between edges and so on, the object can still easily be identified. Though an object presents many different faces we see the same object, and it is by no means easy to accommodate this in any kind of theory trafficking in stimuli and their analysis. The idea that for anything that one can identify there is an invariant property of the array of receptor excitation, and that neuronal networks act to detect and classify such patterns, irrespective of context, does not seem a fruitful view.

It is clear, however, that certain observations, particularly in ethology, can fit well with the idea that some behaviour is organized aorund classification of stimuli, and that these classifications are supported by neuronal classifying networks. This, no doubt, was the kind of evidence that Horridge (1968) had in mind to support the arguments quoted earlier in this chapter. It would be surprising if the behaviour of the tick (von Uexküll, 1934) were supported in any other way, and there are many other invertebrate examples, some of the simpler of which seem well on the way to giving a complete specification of the nervous system of whole animals (e.g. Kandel, 1974).

It may be that there is a difference between invertebrate and vertebrate organization, because in some apparently simple mammalian examples the situation seems to point in rather a different direction. Take again, for example, the problem of discrimination of orientation. The simplest account of how Hubel and Wiesel's (1959, 1962) orientation selective units operate is that simple, complex and hyper-complex cells constitute successively higher levels in a hierarchical classification network. Simple cells receive connections from a set of lateral geniculate cells with concentric receptive fields arranged in a row. Thus the optimal response of a simple cell occurs when all the receptive fields in that row are stimulated, and the cell then acts as a classifier for straight bars or edges. Similarly, the complex cell can be thought of as being connected to a set of simple cells which are all sensitive to a particular orientation and which have adjacent receptive fields. The complex cell responds optimally for a correctly orientated bar, but independently of precise position within the large receptive field of the complex cell. To imagine neural networks performing these functions is quite easy (see e.g. Oatley, 1972 or Lindsay and Norman, 1972), and the step from a cell at one level of the hierarchy to a cell at the next (say, from a simple to a complex cell) requires only one synapse. The more recent extensions of this kind of analysis, e.g. by Stone and Dreher, 1973, make a further classification into separate channels of 'X' and 'Y' neurones which are proposed to subserve sustained form vision, and vision for movements respectively. No doubt, neurophysiologists will continue to be successful in penetrating further and further into the visual system in this way. But when neurones, such as those described by Gross *et al* (1972), specific to a primate hand, or by Updyke (1974) as specific to three-dimensional objects, but not pictures on a screen, are found we are far from understanding either the role of the neurones or the significance of their response properties. Nor could we describe a classification network which had those properties.

Recalling the analogy drawn in the first chapter between recording from a neurone and from an element in the central processor of a computer: an element may respond to a particular stimulus, but this does not mean that the role it is playing in the machine is a classifier of that stimulus. It might also be responsive if it were performing some quite different function. Both for line detectors for which we can imagine an underlying neural network, or for hand detectors, for which we cannot, the interpretation of their properties requires a theory, and the stimulus classification theory may no longer be fruitful.

A further cause for disquiet about the simplistic neurophysiological scheme of classificatory neurones underlying behaviour is that even when the behaviour required of the animal is precisely that of classification, as in a discrimination task, neurones which might seem to be capable of supporting that classification do not seem uncessarily to be involved. Hirsch and Spinelli (1970) reared cats so that all they saw with one eye was a field of horizontal stripes and all they saw with the other was a field of vertical ones. Unit recording from the visual cortex following this early experience revealed that the only orientation sensitive neurones that could be found were those responsive to stimuli, presented to a given eye, which were in an orientation at or near the orientation with which that eye had been reared. Hirsch (1972), having resuscitated a number of these cats after the neurophysiological experiments, found that in discrimination tests the animals were capable of learning discriminations between orientations for which they evidently lacked neurones. Subsequent further neurophysiological testing revealed that this lack still persisted. Although unit recording admittedly samples only a small number of neurones, the results still seem odd: one would expect orientation discriminations to be completely disrupted by such a swingeing loss of orientation sensitive cells as is produced by orientation selective rearing, yet apparently the behavioural deficit, though Hirsch found one, was rather small.

Although no experiments which might be thought to relate electrophysiological properties to behavioural function of (for instance) orientation sensitive neurones allow one completely to reject the idea that these neurones are feature classifiers on the basis of whose activities discriminations might be formed, there are no experiments that give strong support to this notion. One kind of experiment which has been expected to give such support is the adaptation experiment, in which after inspecting stimuli supposedly adequate for a particular class of neurones, subjects show some change in perceptual function or threshold to these stimuli. It seems plausible that such work might throw light on the perceptual significance of particular classes of neurone. Since the idea was first put forward by Sutherland (1961) as an explanation of figural after-effects in terms of adaptation of Hubel and Wiesel's (1959) orientation detectors, and of movement after-effects in terms of adaptation of Barlow and Hill's (1963) movement detectors, such schemes have become widely accepted. If correct, the notion would indicate an involvement of specific classes of cells in perceptual function. But there seem to be differences between psychological adaptation and neuronal adaptation. Whereas the latter may last a few days or even weeks in the case of some contingent after-effects (Mayhew and Anstis, 1972) typical neuronal adaptation times are very much shorter, or longer ones have yet to be discovered.

Moreover, in contingent after-effects, Mayhew and Anstis have found a phenomenon for which they use the Gestalt term transposition, which corresponds with Lashley's statement that we respond not to the particular stimulation, but to relational properties. In one experiment, for instance, observers looked alternatively at a disc rotating clockwise while illuminated with red light, and anticlockwise while illuminated with yellow light. The normal contingent after-effect was found: that is when the stationary disc was illuminated with red or yellow it appeared to rotate in the opposite direction to that during adaptation, i.e. the after-effect was anticlockwise for red, and clockwise for yellow. If, however, the pair of illuminating lights used in the tests were transposed along the spectrum to yellow and green, the movement after-effect was still anticlockwise for the longer wavelength (now yellow, which previously had been the shorter wavelength and which had produced a clockwise after-effect), and clockwise for the shorter wave (green) light. Putting it another way, following adaptation only to red and yellow lights with the two directions of movement, the after-effect to a yellow stationary disc depended on the colour of the previous test light. If immediately preceding the yellow disc the observer had viewed the stationary red disc (as in the adaptation condition), the yellow seemed to move clockwise. However, after viewing a green disc not seen during adaptation the yellow one seemed to move anticlockwise.

It is no easier to square this kind of observation with what we at present know about feature detecting cells in the visual system than it was to understand Lashley's (1938) findings of similar relational transposition in size discriminations, despite the belief that adaptation can be understood as affecting specific feature detecting neurones. The context or relationships of a pattern are evidently all important for how it is seen.

This is not to say that efforts to relate neurophysiological function to behaviour in adaptation experiments have not been informative. They have been, and the subject will be taken up later in chapters 7 and 8. However, although attempts have been made to relate perceptual function to the adequate stimuli of so-called feature detecting neurones, none of these attempts (in mammals at least) seems as such to have been wholly successful within the terms of the theory that neurones are stimulus classifiers. Demonstrable relationships relating neurophysiology to perception are particularly important, since they could provide a link in the chain of explanation of psychology in terms of the workings of the brain. The conclusion from the failure to demonstrate that neurones are simply classifiers that transform an environmental event into a stimulus (within the terms of a stimulus-response theory) is that the notions that neurones are classifying units and that perception is classification are inadequate. Classification filtering and the application of transforms by neural networks on aspects of the receptor array may well go on. Indeed, it seems likely that it does. What seems less likely is that the whole of perception consists entirely of such classification, filtering and transforming of particular patterns in the receptor array.

Lashley's most famous experimental attack on reflex theory was made against the idea of the neural connection. In *Brain Mechanisms and Intelligence* published in 1929 Lashley reported two main types of experiment on the relation of the cortical lesions to rats' performance in mazes. In one type of experiment, cortical lesions of varying size and varying location were made, and the operated rats were compared with normal animals in their learning of mazes of varying difficulty (and also in their learning of other tasks). In the second type of experiment rats first learned a maze, and were then operated upon. These lesioned animals were then compared for retention of the maze habit with unoperated ones which had learned the same task. In these experiments the extent of cortical removal in the lesioned animals ranged from a few per cent to eighty per cent of the total cortex, and in one or other animal in the series, every part of the cortex had been removed.

In the first series, it was found that lesions of the cortex did interfere with rats' abilities to learn mazes, but no particular part of the cortex seemed to affect learning more than any other. Instead, deterioration in learning ability seemed to be a function of the total amount of cortical tissue removed, independently of its locus. In the second, it was found that retention of an already learned maze seemed to be affected in the same way.

These results are, of course, well known. So, at least for many psychology undergraduates, is the nature of the debate that then takes place on the significance of Lashley's work. This debate is well expressed by Zangwill (1961). There is, for instance, the proposition that maze learning is not a well defined task. For better defined tasks the situation may be different. Thus for pattern vision a rather small area of the visual cortex seems to be necessary, and extirpations of other areas have relatively little effect. So there is localization. Subsequently most cortical lesion makers have confined their attention to discovering well defined tasks, and attributing specific behavioural deficits to specific locations of brain lesions. Lashley himself did not deny these findings indeed he himself made several such. A further proposition in the argument, which Lashley did deny, was that the maze habit deteriorated because of the loss of specific sensory capacities attendant upon cortical damage.

Then the undergraduate tries to come to grips with what Lashley really means by 'equipotentiality' and 'mass action'. Equipotentiality was defined by Lashley in 1929 as the 'apparent capacity of any intact part of a functional area to carry out with or without reduction in efficiency the functions which are lost by destruction of the whole'. Mass action he stated is a law 'whereby the efficiency of performance of an entire complex function may be reduced in proportion to the extent of brain injury within an area whose parts are not more specialized for one component of the function than for another'. Evidently, the ideas of a 'function' and a 'functional area' are important. Function seems to mean 'measurable aspect of behaviour' and the conclusion from *Brain Mechanisms and Intelligence* is that the whole cortex is a functional area for maze learning. The occipital cortex is a functional area for brightness discriminations.

Lashley himself paraded a number of possible explanations for his evidence that it was the amount and not the location of the lesion that affected performance. In 1943 he listed six types of explanation: (1) indirect effects of a lesion – such as diaschisis, surgical shock, generalized pressure changes etc.; (2) invasion of areas critical for a particular function; (3) simulated sensory deficits because cortical damage might be equivalent to depriving the animal of sensory modalities; (4) progressive invasion of association areas; (5) interference with interactions between diverse functional areas and (6) a reduced dynamic mass action of the cortex.

It was largely by arguing against explanations one to five that Lashley was left with the residual hypothesis of mass action to explain his results. Few people in brain research have been as good as Lashley at seeing what was wrong with other peoples' theories and hypotheses, so that reading Lashley's arguments one can easily be convinced. But in writing one's undergraduate essay on Lashley one must be critical, and on being critical it becomes clear that Lashley himself in his mass action hypothesis had not much of an explanation to offer. Part of the reason, which can be made either explicitly or implicitly in one's essay is that by the strict criteria which have come to be regarded as necessary in this refractory subject, Lashley was not a good theoretician. His theory of mass action can not easily be tested or refuted. Neither, by these terms, was he a good experimenter. Some of his demonstrations which supposedly showed that this or that function was not localized within some area, or that a particular cortical removal, or a knife cut severing supposed association pathways, did not measurably affect behaviour, were suspiciously like trying to prove the null hypothesis. Such experiments are always liable to attack by someone who uses a better measuring technique. In the rationale of experimenting, a difference between experimental and control groups can have attributed to it a measurable degree of reliability: a probability of the difference occurring by chance being one in twenty, one in a hundred, one in a thousand or whatever. A null result where control and experimental groups score the same has no measurable reliability. It might mean that there really is no difference: but it might mean that if the experimenter had used more subjects or a more sensitive test he would have found one. Thus the 'competent' experimental practitioner casts his theory and experiment into a form that produces differences.

This no doubt is why, although the popularity of brain lesioning as an experimental technique was at least partly due to Lashley's influence, the emphasis has shifted to discovering what functions can be described as localized, because here differences between experimental and control animals can be sought.

Unfortunately, despite experimental orthodoxy, the most striking thing about Lashley's results was precisely that so much brain damage made so little difference to behaviour. Though Lashley more clearly than anyone else in his time saw this as indicating the inadequacies of reflex theory and even of its less obvious but more deeply ingrained concepts, the stimulus, the connection and the response, he had nothing much better to put in its place. Mass action is no kind of explanation of how the brain works. It is simply Lashley's short-hand term for describing his finding that a behavioural deficit depends on the size, not the location of a lesion within a functional area. Thus although Lashley declared himself to be unimpressed 'with analogies between various machines and neural activity' the truth is that he had nothing very substantial to use as an analogy for what the brain was like, that is to say, no better analogy than the Cartesian one, no theory which he could test.

Although the debate over Lashley's results is regarded as an important one in psychology, and central to physiological psychology, it is now rather a muted one. Lashley's mass action work has not really been followed by a stream of further investigations in the same way as has, for instance, Olds and Milner's (1954) discovery of self stimulation. Rather, as I have indicated, lesion makers here turned their attention away and sought 'positive' results, trying precisely to define behavioural deficits attributable to particular lesions.

Yet as Hebb (1963) remarks in his introduction to the reprint of *Brain Mechanisms and Intelligence*, in the few years following the first appearance of this monograph psychology changed from a subject in which there was an easy assumption that a relation between stimulus and response was mediated by a neural pathway, that a memory was located in a single neurone, and so on, to a conspicuous avoidance of such neurologizing. Before Lashley, theorizing in psychology tended to be physiological, afterwards many psychologists declared themselves only to be competent to discuss 'functional' relationships between stimuli and responses, and not their neural embodiments.

What happened seemed to be that Lashley had achieved a refutation of reflex theory, albeit one that was experimentally not very satisfactory. But because there was not anything much better to put in its place, psychologists continued to talk about stimuli and responses thereby retaining the thinking of the old theory, and simply avoiding the mention of connections as such. Physiological psychologists turned to studying such matters as lesion produced behavioural deficits such as the failure of rats to eat following a lesion in the lateral hypothalamus (Hetherington and Ranson, 1940) or the issue of what behavioural components actually suffer with a lesion. (It is somewhat curious that now even the apparently rather specific properties of various subcortical areas investigated in the last thirty-five years seem not to be so specific, see e.g. Valenstein, 1973.)

But without any alternatives the tacit theory that stimuli and response are somehow to be connected in the brain continued. Learning, for instance, is still seen as a higher process, but one that within the theory can only really be conceptualized as understanding how a stimulus becomes associated with an appropriate response.

The prize of 'understanding learning' beckons strongly, and the psychologist continues in his quest with the quick sidestep of concerning himself not with neural connecting pathways, but the logical structure of the associative process. The physiologist sidesteps in the other direction. Even if pathways between stimulus and response cannot be assumed, changes in nervous system must still take place in learning. Since neuronal mechanisms seem to work in terms of connections between neurones, where else is there for change to take place except at the synapses? Thus the search for the physiological basis of learning is directed towards the synapse, and again despite the sidestep, the pervading theory exhorts us to believe that the way towards understanding behaviour is in terms of a connection between stimulus and response.

This latter search ranges over changes in protein synthesis brought about by altered RNA molecules, to changes in transmitter metabolism or electrical properties in neural tissue as a function of the preceding stimulation, and the findings are by no means without interest. However, they no more carry the possibility of revealing the secret of learning than did the discoveries of how nerve impulses were transmitted revealed how the brain works. In all likelihood a large number of neural processes will be discovered to act as storage progesses. Adaptation (as described by Adrian, 1928) which allows a receptor to compare the current level of input with the (remembered) just previous one, and so transmit a signal corresponding to the rate of change of some parameter, is an example discovered a long time ago, and there is good reason to believe (see e.g. the discussion on learning in this chapter) that many other neural processes have storage properties of particular kinds.

However, the real point is that storage, or memory in the sense that a computer is sometimes said to have memory in magnetic core store, is not necessarily a complex process. It is indeed a common, even a banal process. A scratch on a table where I cut a slice of bread without using a plate or a breadboard is a memory of that event. A physical change has taken place to the table which will store or record, more or less permanently, the occurrence of that event. It is that kind of change which is being referred to in discussions of the physiological basis of memory.

But if I were to see a scratch on a table and interpret it as an indication of an event that occurred when someone was cutting a slice of bread, I could only reconstruct that event if I happened to know about bread, and serrated breadknives, the conventions of behaviour in that type of household and many other things. Without a theory about domestic arrangements and utensils in the kind of house where the table was, no one would be able to interpret the mark on the table, or 'remember', that is to say reconstruct, the actual event. This example may not be a bad metaphor for human memory. It is not the process of storage, the physical change produced by an event, that is difficult to understand. That indeed is rather trivial. It is the organization of such stored signs and their interpretation which are difficult to comprehend. As Bartlett (1932) made clear, human memory is a reconstructive process, i.e. a process such as concluding that someone made the scratch on a table by carelessly cutting bread. Understanding how such a rich complex set of cultural knowledge is brought to bear on stored events is a difficult problem, and one which has rather little to do with stimulus-response connections.

Putting this another way, just as understanding the nature of the change made on the paper by the ink that is used to print these words is irrelevant to understanding how it is possible to leave a permanent record (memory?) of thoughts, so understanding the nature of the physiological event that allows storage of information may be largely irrelevant to understanding human or animal memory. This is not to say that the invention of printing is unimportant. Far from it. But what allows one to leave a record of thoughts is principally the knowledge of language which both writer and reader must possess, and the symbolic properties of writing. Thus when one speaks of memory or learning one is not speaking simply of some semi-permanent change in brain cells, but of an organization of symbolic processes which allows the brain to represent a state of the world and also allows interpretation of that information subsequently so that the information may come meaningfully to influence thoughts and/or behaviour.

The quality of stimulus-response theory is to make an identification of the problems of learning (or memory) with that of storage is instrumental in reaching the conclusion that understanding the physiological basis of storage will lead us to a comprehension of higher nervous processes. If it would not be rubbing the point in too much the following seems to be the kind of argument that displays this identification. John (1967) for instance writes

> Whatever we have come to know of the brain it has remained difficult to understand how mind arises from brain. It is perhaps the challenge of this age-old riddle that makes the study of memory so compelling. For, whatever the nature of the storage and retrieval of information in the brain, when we retrieve information we may become aware of it ... Somewhere in the processes that generate remembering must lie in a clue to the processes that generate the most

remarkable feature of our brains — our subjective experience.

Following this argument the next stage is to define learning, since if we can do that satisfactorily, we will be able to study examples of the process in animals, determine how its physiological, biophysical and biochemical bases give rise to the behaviour called learning, and we are then in the business of understanding the mind.

At this point one may come to the embarrassing conclusion that discoveries of certain kinds of neural storage have not thrown a blinding light on the nature of our most valued mental states. For this reason a definition of learning which would be judged satisfactory must be one which captures the rather exalted status of what we normally take to be the 'important' psychological phenomenon of learning, while at the same time excluding changes which seem to be rather trivial. As Booth (1970) has pointed out, there is a certain odd contortion in this type of attempt: for instance a typical textbook definition might hold that 'learning is behavioural change that is not caused by growth, maturation, degeneration, damage, environmental variation, or behavioural variability attributable to cyclic or random internal changes.' The strange forms such definitions take seem to indicate that those who offer the definitions believe that learning is too complex and subtle for us to accept that it can be classed with phenomena such as fatigue or growth. In constructing an acceptable definition, therefore, there seems, amongst other things, to be an attempt to guard against the possibility that some too simple process should be acceptable as the basis of learning. Then the concept of 'Grade A Certified Learning' which these definitions try to capture is reached.

The common element in all the matters to which psychologists and physiologists seem to be referring when they discuss learning and memory is in fact storage. But, as I have indicated, storage can be an extremely simple, even a trivial operation with nothing strange or difficult about it (cf. the punched hole in the computer card). Clearly complex and subtle phenomena, such as how we learn to dress ourselves, or how we remember the face of a friend, are not explained by understanding how storage occurs; though they might be by understanding the organization of logical operations which manipulate and interpret the stored information. It is only within theories which state that learning is the root of man's highest faculties, and consists of the acquisition of new connections, or change in the probability of response, that the issue of whether the discovery of a storage process could solve the 'age-old riddle' of how mind arises from brain needs to be raised.

As to responses, Lashley was again at work. Lashley and McCarthy (1926) showed that rats subjected to cerebellar injuries after they had learned a maze could still traverse the maze without errors, even though their gait was grossly impaired and that in order to reach the goal box the animals had to execute a series of movements which were very different than those used when they learned the task.

In 1942 Lashley showed a rather good picture (fig. 4.4) of writing performed by various muscle groups, with the pen held in either hand, with a foot, and in the mouth. The pattern is

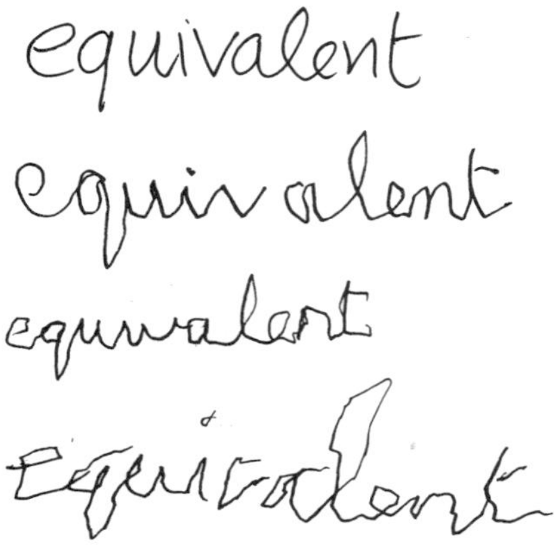

Figure 4.4 Response equivalence (from an idea of Lashley 1942): the word 'equivalent' written respectively with a pen held in the right hand, left hand, mouth, and right foot.

preserved, despite the complete difference of the muscles or indeed the 'movements' involved. 'Motor habits', he concluded, 'are no more rigidly restricted to a small number of specialized cellular elements than is sensory perception.'

In his famous paper on serial order in behaviour of 1951 Lashley discussed how within reflex theory one assumes that a skilled action consists of a series of movements, in which each sensory result, or feedback from each component, triggers off the next. This can also be called a reflex chain theory: the first element would be triggered off by some external stimulus and each response would produce an event which stimulates the next. The reason why this kind of idea cannot in general serve as a theory of how motor elements are organized into specific sequences is most clearly illustrated by language. Even if words were to be classified as individual movements (itself too simple a notion), then the problem of how we could speak a sentence with a given order of words cannot be solved by supposing that elements trigger each other reflexly. If this were the case, we would get in a hopeless muddle trying to construct a sentence such as 'The millwright on my right thinks it right that some conventional rite should symbolize the right of every man to write as he pleases.' Yet Lashley managed both to construct the sentence and speak it. Clearly word order cannot in any sense be determined by direct associations of the word 'right' with any others, but (perhaps) by meaning and grammar.

Lashley also pointed out that feedback from proprioceptive or other sensory sources was too slow to be important in many types of motor performance: in playing musical instruments it would be no good waiting for the sound or the proprioceptive accompaniment of having played a note in order to know when to begin the next. Reaction time would limit the highest rate of note playing to four or five a second, whereas skilled musicians can play at rates of up to sixteen notes per second.

And so it goes on. One could get the impression that Lashley in a long and very full research life was obsessed with showing that reflexes did not provide an adequate basis for understanding behaviour.

Besides his attacks on stimuli, connections, and responses Lashley had some pertinent things to say about the doctrine of levels and the elevation of learning to a pre-eminent place. Take, for instance, the idea that the intelligent behaviour of our own large brains is based on learning, whereas lower animals with less developed brains depend on instinct. This as Lashley (1949) pointed out is palpably false. Many lowly animals such as worms can under favourable conditions learn a simple association in a single trial. More recently it has been shown that even animals as lowly as coelenterates (Ross, 1965) and flatworms (Thompson and McConnell, 1955) can be classically conditioned. Moreover, although there are two major orders of advanced insects, the flies on one hand and the wasps, bees and ants on the other, flies only with difficulty learn anything (in experimental situations at least). Bees and wasps on the other hand perform quite impressive feats of learning. For example, the digger wasp circles the entrance to a burrow where she has laid an egg for a few seconds before setting off to find a bee to put in the hole as a store of food for her larva, and learns during this brief circling the surrounding landmarks of twigs and stones (Tinbergen, 1951).

Nor are the lowest vertebrates entirely dim. A tropical goby fish studied by Aaronson (1956) often gets trapped in a rock pool when the tide goes out. If disturbed in this situation, the fish will jump out of its pool into a neighbouring pool, nearly always avoiding landing on intervening rocks. Indeed it can hop to the sea via a number of pools. Placed in a novel set of rock pools these fish do not jump accurately, but in one of Aaronson's experiments, after the fish were allowed a single twelve-hour period of artificial high tide in an artificial set of rock pools, they were able to jump accurately. By contrast there is serious question (which was accompanied by a dispute raging in the psychological literature for several years, see e.g. Kimble, 1961) whether the rat, a higher mammal, could perform this kind of so-called latent learning task at all (digger wasps and gobies certainly can). In navigational ability, which includes learning of landmarks (e.g. Matthews, 1955), the pigeon with only a stunted homologue of a cortex performs in a way that is certainly comparable to that of humans. (Actually people's navigational abilities when they are not relying on artificial instruments are also quite impressive, see e.g. Oatley, 1974, though no direct contest seems yet to have been staged.)

Furthermore mammals do depend heavily on instinctive, that is to say genetically specified mechanisms. The nervous system is 'not a natural medium on which learning imposes any form of organization whatever' (Lashley, 1949).

It is, for instance, quite easy to learn to discriminate the patterns on the left of fig. 4.5, but extremely difficult for either rats or people to discriminate between the patterns on the right. To give just one other example here, Chomsky (e.g. 1968) has pointed out that one very characteristically human behaviour, speech, seems to require substantial innate basis. Although the actual language a child acquires is obviously learned, both the fact that a child can learn a language at all, and the fact that even though his or her experience of specific

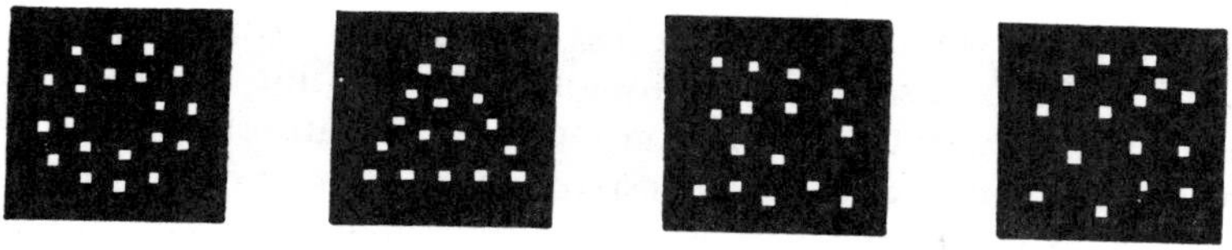

Figure 4.5 Structured and unstructured arrangements of dots. Both people and rats find it easy to recognise the patterns on the left and difficult to recognise the patterns on the right (from Lashley, 1949).

linguistic utterances is both fragmentary and disjointed, he or she nevertheless becomes capable of producing entirely novel sentences which are nonetheless meaningful and grammatical. It seems unreasonable to suppose that this would be possible if there did not exist brain mechanisms capable of allowing an interpretation of sounds the infant hears, and incorporation of their neural counterparts into pre-existing structures that form the basis of grammar. The elaborate and painstaking recent efforts to teach chimpanzees language (e.g. Premack, 1971) do not contradict this point. As a colleague pointed out to me, they are rather like the attempt to teach an elephant to climb trees. We might be very impressed when after many reinforced trials the elephant was able to grasp an overhanging branch with its trunk, and place its front feet on the tree, but is that climbing?

There is no point in reviewing here in greater detail either arguments or evidence of the inadequacy of reflex theory or its ramifications to explain most behaviour. Arguments have a well-known potential for fallibility and even an experimental result of any kind is not really a fact, or evidence against a particular theory. It is a datum which can be more or less well interpreted within a given theory. If it is shown that it is not the particular set of receptor elements that is important in perception, then within reflex theory the conclusion could be that stimuli are more complex than we thought.

To return to the example of the first chapter, a chair is referred to as visual stimulus despite the fact that there are no retinal criteria for classifying all chairs. There is no set of visual patterns which define the conception 'chair'. A chair is an artificial object with surfaces to support the body when sitting, and it is these functional criteria which allow us to recognize it when we see it. Yet the words visual stimulus continue to be used. Neurophysiologists continue to look for neurones with more and more complex 'adequate stimuli', as if even when a neurone which responded to a chair or a grandmother, it would tell us anything about how the recognition was achieved. It would not. We know that behaviourally we can recognize chairs and even occasionally grandmothers. To call these stimuli, and announce that there is some neurophysiological event which corresponds to stimulus classification is to say rather little except to demonstrate an adherence to the theoretical proposition that there are stimuli, and the idea that identifying adequate stimuli completes the process of understanding vision.

As far as connections between stimulus and response go, again if direct simple pathways cannot be discovered, this need not be a signal to abandon reflex theory. The theory can be retained and its adherents simply stop thinking about what a connection is like as Skinner (1938) suggests, while still studying the properties of these connections. Alternatively, one can suppose that the physiological connections exist, but that they are more complex and subtle than was thought. Thus, for instance, in 1949 Lashley's student, Hebb, put forward a theory to explain stimulus equivalence and Lashley's (1929) failure in cortical extirpation experiments to localize any regions in which the memories were located. Hebb's suggestion was that the neural connections were structural but plentiful and diffuse.

The problem of response equivalence is similar to that of stimulus equivalence, and adhering to reflex theory the answer could be the same. A response is more complex than one might think. In fact the complicated nature of a response even in supposedly simple reflexes has been recognized for many years, certainly by Hughlings Jackson. The motor system is organized to produce not muscular contractions but purposive actions, independently of particular circumstances. Thus withdrawal of the hand from flame which happens to be on a match we are holding might involve a pattern of muscular contractions which is quite different from those which would occur if the flame were on a gas stove we had inadvertently touched. One can, of course, call the action a response and the whole behavioural event a withdrawal reflex. Setting out along this path one soon finds oneself with Pavlov (1927) talking about the investigatory reflex, the freedom reflex and so forth. Purposeful actions seem to be categorized as responses simply in order to give them a meaning which stimulus response analysis can handle.

Assessing the weight of recent neurophysiological knowledge about which he is acknowledgedly erudite, Horridge (1969) concluded in favour of the reflex theory of behaviour.

According to Horridge (as discussed previously) all interneurones are units of pattern recognition, that is to say, classificatory elements. The final result of such classifications are behavioural responses, or choices as he calls them, and the repertoire of these is very limited. 'Apart from facts of human memory, and the specialized actions of primates and a few other mammals such as elephants, an act of behaviour in an experimental test of a cat, rat, octopus or crab is relatively simple. The total number of choices described in all psychological literature could be punched on comparatively few yards of tape'. What is involved (says Horridge) is that certain types of stimulus pattern classified as such by banks of interneurones trigger the output of particular motor patterns selected from the small number available. Behaviour is explained.

Lashley's experimentation was in some sense a series of demonstrations that many people suffered from oversimplification in their attempts to understand the brain, and he continued to offer experimental evidence that it was more complicated than people thought. Yet there seems no point in attacking the reflex formulation, or the idea of a hierarchy of higher levels watching over the reflex connections and controlling them out of superior wisdom, with still more mere evidence.

Since Descartes we have in psychology and neurophysiology been practising what Kuhn (1962) calls 'normal science', that is science within the framework of an accepted theoretical framework. That framework has articulated the questions of how stimuli are received by receptors, how neural messages are transmitted, what the neural switching operations are like. It has also given us the issue of learning (how new connections are formed) and the genesis of the work in perception which asks how auditory, tactile and visual patterns are recognized. All this has been useful.

One present-day conclusion could be that the conceptual elements of the theory are more complex than had been thought. But is this an ad hoc patching up? The paradigm, or as Lakatos (1970) calls it the research programme which was successful and productive may have become degenerative. But, within a research programme which is making ad hoc alterations to its theoretical structure, such alterations can occasionally transform the structure sufficiently to convert it again into a progressive fruitful programme. In other words, people working within a paradigm not only tend not to see it as degenerative, but they might be right in patching it up to give it a new lease of life. This, perhaps, is what those people are doing who say that certainly they do not entertain reflex theory, and are not impressed with the stimulus-response formulation, but who continue nevertheless to use the words stimulus and response, or who try to discover the laws or relations or associations between them, and who work to give the concepts better meanings.

However, during the process of assimilating the ideas that stimuli, connections and responses are more complex or subtle than we thought, the criterion of the reflex as a workable mechanism has been relaxed. If stimuli can be anything that we can see; trees, monsters, affectionate looks, handwritten sentences etc., and responses can range across smiling, writing a novel, feeling depressed, kicking a football etc., we are quite unable to specify a reflex mechanism that would perform these. Thus the criterion that the mechanism of the theory can produce something corresponding to behaviour is no longer met. But the reflex maintains its aura of being explanatory, because it has been displayed as a mechanism, despite the fact that with any modifications substantial enough to meet the experimental evidence of Lashley and others, it just will not work. If it were to be made to work, and continued to be the dominant and progressive theoretical notion, brain research might be a pretty dull subject, with the only major theoretical principle the reflex, and that discovered 300 years ago. (Perhaps this is why undergraduates who embark upon psychology courses with high hopes, rather soon start to feel that there is something about academic psychology that does not live up to their expectations.) Of course, there can be subsidiary theories explaining how sensory patterns were classified, how responses were made up and so forth. But the only basic theory would be the reflex.

Fortunately this seems unlikely to be the case. Old theoretical schemes do not continue, they tend to fade slowly and become irrelevant when better ones appear. We have probably been stuck with stimuli and responses because of the lack of anything better with which to compare the brain than hydraulically operated statues, telephone systems and the like. A new paradigm may now be appearing in which potentially we have a whole set of much more powerful metaphors derived from artificial devices which for the first time do exhibit something of the flexibility, versatility and complexity of symbol manipulation that the brain has. Armed with better concepts, new kinds of theory, which do not refute the old, but which allow the data to be seen in, perhaps, a more productive way, are beginning to emerge.

Carrying the notion of paradigms and revolutionary changes in scientific theory a little further, both neurophysiology and experimental psychology still have something of the character of Aristotelian physics. Greek physics essentially translated our naive understandings of physical phenomena into something that had the flavour of mechanism. People commonly observed that objects fell downwards. Movement was, therefore, explained as objects being attracted towards their natural resting place, the centre of the earth. If terrestrial objects moved in any other way, e.g. an arrow through the air or a ball rolling across a flat surface, then they must be continuously propelled by a force, just as a person has continually to propel a handcart or the wind to blow a square-rigged ship. Celestial bodies, observed to execute circular motions round the earth, evidently move in a different and indeed more perfect way: the explanation being that they are fixed to celestial spheres rotating around their centre, the earth. In each case the explanation has the flavour of mechanism, (or perhaps one should say 'animism') but it is scarcely more than a description of what is observed: the arrow is propelled by a force which keeps it flying in the air, the planet executes a circular orbit because it is fixed to a sphere (with circular cross section) rotating about its centre.

Descartes' theory of the reflex did better than to give the flavour of mechanism. The metaphor or analogy he used of hydraulically operated statues was a real mechanism, and the neural embodiment of that has been the subject of fruitful research. But in the question of what stimuli and responses are, again there is little more than redescription of naive observation.

To explain how the same end is achieved by a variety of motor means, we call a purposeful action a response. To explain how we can recognize a dog, a friend, a church designed by Hawksmoor, a thunderstorm on its way, or a film that we have seen before, we can call each of these a stimulus. Furthermore, we then do experiments in which we use prototypical stimuli, patches of light, patterns of lines carefully fixated, sinusoidal gratings etc. We can then change parameters of these patches of light projected onto the retina, and since these changes clearly alter the stimulus conditions, we can believe that we collect facts about the conditions of perception. Our experiments are ones in which we tend to create data relevant to the theory of stimuli and responses.

What the reflex theory lacks as Aristotelian physics lacked is something going on beneath the superficial appearances of phenomena that would give them the qualities they seem to have. In both cases the supposed mechanism was supposed simply to have the quality sufficient to do what was observed. A force is defined as that which is capable of keeping the arrow in the air. A visual stimulus is that pattern of stimulation arising from a particular object or event which provokes a response.

Kuhn (1957) describes how Hooke in 1666 demonstrated to the Royal Society a weight on the end of a piece of string. When displaced from its point of rest, the forces acting on the weight attracted it towards its original position, with the string hanging exactly vertically. But when propelled in any direction not through this point the weight took up an eliptical orbit around it, the nature of the elipse depending on the way the weight was propelled. This was a model of planetary motion. Better known than Hooke's demonstration is, of course, Newton's treatment of two forces, acting at right angles to each other, gravitational and inertial, which give rise to the family of circular and eliptical orbits, and parabolic trajectories of arrows. An observed circular orbit is not now explained by the operation of something circular, but as an emergent property of the interaction of unobserved processes with a different character. It is exactly this notion of the emergent properties of behaviour and mental processes arising from quite different operations of the brain which is missing from so many explanations in physiology and physiological psychology, and particularly from explanations in terms of stimuli, connections and responses.

5 *Emergent properties*

In one of Molière's plays a doctor, on being asked why opium made one sleepy, explained earnestly that the opium worked by means of its 'dormitive potency'. Despite this subterfuge several hundred years ago, the rather similar process of mapping descriptions or categories of behaviour on to regions of the brain (e.g. sleep is controlled by a sleep centre) seems widely accepted today. So does the notion that to see an object, say a potato, we consign the retinal image pattern of that potato to the response class of potatoes. Maybe the idea that, if we know the name of some thing, or some process, or some person, we have power over them runs deep.

What we need, in order to escape from this rather fruitless name-dropping, is some understanding of emergent properties; an understanding which will also have another important property of lifting us out of the fallacy that if we comprehend the properties of the fundamental units of a system then we can deduce the properties of the whole: as if each part contained a little bit of the essence of the whole. This, for instance, seems to be the reasoning behind the view of consciousness that it is present in imperceptible or sub-threshold qualities in simple organisms, and when enough complexity is reached the quantity of consciousness reaches a threshold whereupon the system in question becomes conscious.

An understanding of emergent properties also allows us to parry what is now called radical behaviourism. The most vigorous proponent of a grand system of behaviourism is still B.F. Skinner. Skinner claims that his formulation of the problem goes significantly beyond the Cartesian reflex. In a recent book (1972) Skinner is quite clear about the nature of his task. It is to abolish the notion of 'autonomous man' who is conceived of having a mind, and to whom we might attribute such processes as 'understanding'. 'So far as a science of behaviour is concerned autonomous means miraculous', says Skinner. Autonomous man 'is a centre from which behaviour emanates. He initiates, originates and creates and in so doing he remains, as he was for the Greeks, divine.'

Skinner asserts that he has escaped both from the strait-jacket of the Cartesian reflex formulation, and from mystical explanations. He makes the rather striking claim that his system is the first worthwhile advance since Descartes' formulation which, he argues, impeded progress for a long time, because it carried the implication that the environment is a goad (the translation of the Latin stimulus) which forces the organism into action. He replaces it with the idea that the environment acts more subtly by selecting aspects of behaviour which the organism emits. Skinner argues that behaviour is obviously entirely determined by two factors; a genetic endowment and the influence of the environment on the individual. The genetic heritage has come about by a process of evolution in which the environment has acted subtly to select certain spontaneously occurring mutations. In just the same way the process of reinforcement acts inconspicuously to select aspects of behaviour emitted by the individual. Clearly then, the object of psychology is to understand the laws of this environmental process of reinforcement-based selection.

Skinner claims in other words to have discovered some property of the behavioural process which will demystify 'autonomous man', and cope with those processes of perception, understanding and so on which seem so difficult to comprehend.

Skinner's claim seems to rest upon two foundations: first, that behaviour must in some sense derive entirely from genetic capacity and the influence of the environment on the individual, and, secondly, that it can be scientifically studied and explained. Few scientists would question these assumptions. But Skinner's second foundation includes the hidden clause that the influence of the environment is to be investigated using an experimental analysis of behaviour, in which the direct relatedness of environmental cause to behavioural effect is supposedly demonstrated. According to Skinner, it is just this analysis which has deposed autonomous man and his collection of miraculous powers.

On closer examination this experimental analysis of behaviour is found to consist of (a) the demonstration of 'lawful' dependence of some aspects of behaviour of (mainly) rats and pigeons in Skinner boxes on reinforcing and discriminative stimuli, and (b) the assertion that the laws discovered in this context generalize universally to all behaviour of all higher animals. This wider generality is supported by instances such as the following. In a collection of findings on the experimental analysis of behaviour (Verhave, 1966) we are invited to consider how appreciation of music occurs: preferences for modern music were increased by playing modern music while subjects ate a free meal (Razran, 1938). On the subject of linguistic communication reinforcement in the form of the experimenter saying 'Mmmm-Hmmm' when plural words were uttered increased the frequency of plurals spoken by the subject (Greenspoon, 1955). Unfortunately as with any other formulation consisting only of reinforcing stimuli and responses, experimental demonstrations on music or language could scarcely be of any other kind.

Despite Skinner's assertions, autonomous man has not been deposed, merely ignored. In his berating of the notion of autonomous man as unscientific, Skinner is still stuck with a stimulus-response notion of mechanism. Today we can construct devices working according to quite ordinary physical ('scientific') principles that are autonomous; machines that display purpose, machines that in some sense display understanding, and so on. It is absolutely true that such machines are affected by their environment and are indeed responsive to it (and herein lies their interest). But to confine oneself to describing them in terms of stimulus-response relationships would be infinitely laborious and miss some important point. Asserting that mental characteristics (autonomy, understanding) and so on are not comprehensible in terms of relationships between stimulus and response, and, therefore, must be regarded either as magical or non-existent does not make these mental characteristics go away. It merely effectively prevents a system based only on stimuli and responses from being able to say much of significance about these (extensive) areas of man's capacities.

For all these, and no doubt other, reasons we need to know how properties which seem mysterious can emerge from mechanism. As Lorenz (1969) pointed out evolution, despite its name, is not just an unfolding of what was already there, it is the creation of something entirely new, albeit from old elements. Lorenz chooses an example of emergence of new properties from electronic circuits. A simple circuit consisting of a capacitor and a resistor will respond exponentially to a sudden change of voltage (see fig. 5.1a), so too will an inductor (a coil) with a resistor (see fig. 5.1b). However, these same elements can be put together into another circuit, and an entirely new behaviour will be produced, an oscillation (see fig. 5.1c). In this case the oscillation dies gently away following

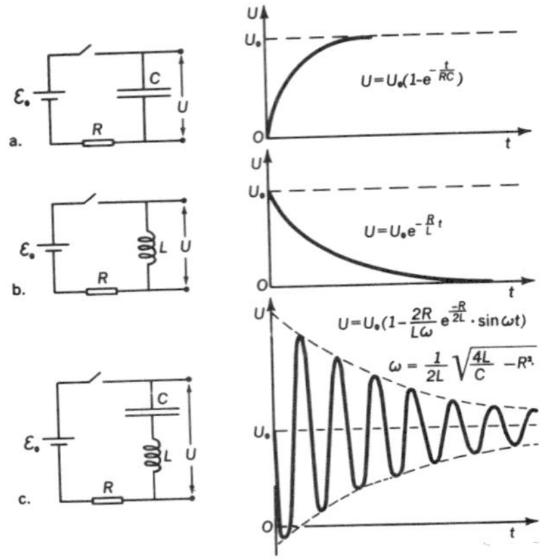

Figure 5.1 Emergent properties: diagram to illustrate how the property of oscillation emerges from a circuit (c) which combines the elements of two circuits (a) and (b) which do not in themselves produce oscillation (from Lorenz, 1969).

the input step, but there is no question but that the oscillation is an entirely novel property of this circuit. In no sense was the oscillatory potentiality implicitly present in the circuits of fig. 5.1a or b (any more than it is particularly helpful to think of a germ of consciousness being present in a certain atom). The new property emerges not from the properties of the parts themselves, but from a new organization of inter-relations between these parts. This is some of the meaning of the whole being more than the sum of its parts. The notion 'sum' expresses an aggregation, or collection of parts with no particular order or organization. It does not express a structure of inter-relationships between the parts. It is this structure which confers the new properties.

Nor is it necessarily the case that properties emerge as complexity increases. Oscillatory behaviour which does not die away is produced in a circuit, which like the circuits a and b, has only two electronic components, a capacitor and an inductance, but no resistor. The conclusion is that ideas like 'sum' or 'greater complexity', which simply express numerical increases, do not express how a particular structure of inter-relationships will generate particular kinds of behaviour. To do that we need a theory of a structural kind, a theory of the behaviour and properties of systems, not just of components.

Lorenz makes the apposite point that nature has invented new systems; but invented them out of existing parts. Evolution in part means the process of invention: invention carried out by making new combinations of components. Continual improvements of inventions also occur because there is nothing like having constructed something for the first time, to be able to do it better next time. The question of whether the new combinations are invented chancewise, by natural selection of mutations, is not germane to the argument.

Two of the most interesting early attempts to invent relatively formal conceptual systems more productive than those of the simple innate or conditioned reflex, and from which important 'new' features of behaviour could emerge were due to Grindley. In 1927 for instance he pointed out that chain reflexes and other associationistic notions fail to explain purposiveness, since two of the marks of purposiveness were the pursuit of particular goals, and the cessation of that pursuit when the goals were attained. He proposed, therefore, a set of neural elements which he called E cells whose activity was not dependent on external stimulation, but represented particular goals. Purposive behaviour (including thinking) Grindley then supposed was dependent upon what he called 'double innervation' from the E cell system, and from external stimulation. Thus activity would continue, by trial and error, or perhaps in some other fashion until the goal was reached, and some signal of the attainment of this goal (e.g. food, solution of a problem etc) would turn off the E cell activity.

In 1932 Grindley pursuing his ideas (which in retrospect clearly had the quality of ruminations on the subject of feedback), reported the following rather quaint experiment. Four guinea pigs, called Jim, Henry, Tom and Roger, learned to turn their heads to one side (say left) in return for a piece of carrot when a buzzer sounded. Subsequently, the experimenter rewarded the guinea pigs for turning the head to the right, rather than to the left, when the buzzer sounded; and a reversal of the original response was achieved.

Grindley did this experiment to question the assumption that all learning is fundamentally of the conditioned reflex type. The assumption had been that the alternative to this formulation, the law of effect, was only demonstrated in situations of some complexity, where the precise set of conditioned reactions had not been worked out (again the argument from complexity). But Grindley's experiment had a structure that he claimed was as simple as any Pavlovian conditioning experiment, and yet demonstrated that a mechanism in which an indifferent stimulus came to elicit the effect of an inborn reflex could not account for his finding. In particular, the reversal of head turning was achieved not by changing the stimulus situation at all, merely by giving the carrot for a turn of the head to the right rather than the left. The reward seemed to act retrospectively, and something like Thorndike's law of effect seemed to be needed in addition to Pavlov's theory of conditioning.

Thus, as well as producing the first experiment on 'operant conditioning', Grindley seems to have been seeking for principles in which the 'feedback' consequences of behaviour would affect behaviour. These principles required new concepts of organizational structure; not just further complexity of concatenated reflex pathways.

Lorenz's discussion of emergent properties of feedback organization continues along the lines of Grindley's (1932) experiment, with the idea that the novel mechanism of the law-of-effect is equivalent to speeding up evolution (the idea also taken up by Skinner, see above). As well as the trial and error strategy of genetic mutations being met occasionally with the feedback of success of survival, behavioural attempts which are successful are also retained but by the individual.

My view is that we do not really understand this kind of learning, despite its having been studied for many years, because it is not really of a simple 'trial and error' kind, nor is the notion 'reinforcement' as simple as it seems. That is to say, in animal or human behaviour trials are not chosen randomly, or in some simple exhaustive pattern, or in any way that we can yet characterize formally. Rather animals and people deploy highly structured strategies for solving problems that confront them, and if one of these fails, they do not simply select the next response on the list. Learning takes place not simply as the emission of a new response when an error occurs. Rather it involves understanding the particular structure of the mistake and deciding what to do next. What changes is not just the probability of response but the particular hypothesis or theory about the world that we were entertaining when the mistake was made. Thus, though learning by the law of effect is a fundamentally important example of an emergent property, we cannot yet express the nature of the system from which it emerges. Minimally it seems the system would need to be one which would operate with some representation or schema of the environment, or if one prefers, entertain hypotheses about the structure of the relevant environment. From this schema (which includes its current goals) it generates strategies and modifies the schema or the strategies in some structured way on analysis of a failure. (These topics will be discussed further in chapters 6 and 9.)

REGULATORY STRUCTURES

Though the feedback of learning is more important, the feedback involved in certain types of regulated behaviour, including some kinds of motivatied behaviour such as hunger and thirst as expressed in Grindley's (1927) example is, for the present, more comprehensible. As usual, Lashley had something to say on this. He argued (1938) that the discovery by Lorente de No (1933) of recurrent pathways, i.e. loops in neuronal networks, 'perhaps capable of indefinite reverberation', might account for the sustained nature of motivational states. After all, he argues, 'the rat in the maze does not stop running between hunger pangs.' Reverberatory circuits thus might serve the same function as Grindley's E cells of maintaining a central neural drive state until a goal is reached.

Lashley certainly has something in the notion that the loop is an organizational structure fundamentally different from the straight pathway of the reflex, and from which new properties might emerge. However, the course of our understanding of the fundamental structure of motivational mechanisms has taken a somewhat different turn from that envisaged by Lashley: the properties that we understand to have emerged from recurrent loops are mostly of another kind.

Two emergent properties of the feedback loop have become evident in relatively simple kinds of behaviour, the properties of regulation and endogenous rhythmicity. Both of these are basic to behaviour, so that it is possible to see how new properties do emerge, or perhaps are invented or created out of old elements.

One of the simplest examples of regulatory properties

emerging from a particular structured arrangement of elements is the so-called pupillary light reflex. Described as a reflex it has, as one would expect from the theory, the elements of receptor, connecting pathway, and effector. The receptor element is clearly some (or all) of the photoreceptors in the retina, the pathway involves the optic nerve, a branch from it to the midbrain, and some nerves of the parasympathetic division of the autonomic nervous system. The effector is the iris muscle. According to theory, one would expect the reflex to work by light falling on the receptors, the signal being transmitted via the connection path to the iris to make it constrict. For this reflex, we allow that the response is graded; that is the more light, the greater the constriction. We can imagine, for simplicity, that constriction of the pupil is against the opposing, spring-like, force of the sympathetic innervation tending to dilate the pupil.

The pupillary light reflex so described conforms closely to Descartes' specification. The three principal elements are there, and the particular response depends upon the particular connection 'according to the whim of the engineer who made it.' However, with a single and simple change, not to the elements in the system, but to our conception of the signal connections between them, the system is transformed, and acquires a set of novel properties. The change from the notion of the conventional reflex pathway, is, of course, the feedback connection from the iris to the retina. And in this case it was there all the time because as the iris contracts it diminishes the light stimulation falling on the receptors.

Clearly with a graded reflex pathway, if the receptor were entirely uninfluenced by the effector one could establish control of pupil size appropriate to the light. This would be what is known as an open loop control system (see fig. 5.2a). Specifying the signal strength in the connection (e.g. impulse rate in a group of fibres) will specify the pupil size if the whole mechanism is under stable conditions. It is extremely useful to lump the various functions into conceptual components, and to express this system in a language not of specifics, but of information: signals and operations upon them, as in fig. 5.2b. There the receptor function is defined as comparison of the light signal with a standard, and giving an error signal which is the difference between the light signal and standard. The circle with a cross in it is the formal systems symbol for the operation of addition on incoming signals according to the signs given. Comparison (as could be performed by a non-adapting neural receptor) is in these terms, simply a subtraction, so that the error signal is a measure of any difference in

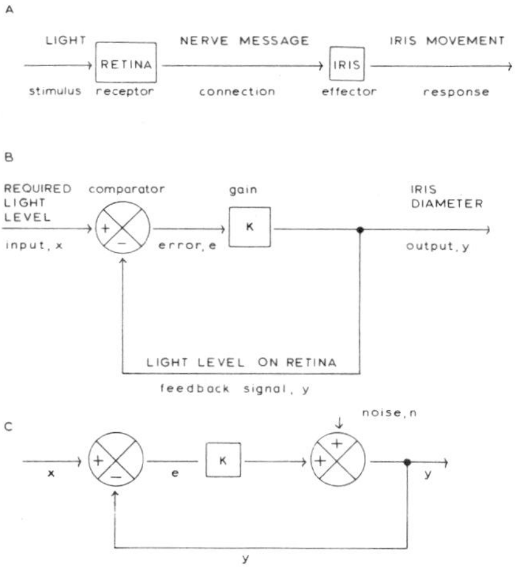

Figure 5.2 Control systems of different kinds: (*a*) *open loop, or reflex control, of the iris,* (*b*) *closed loop, feedback control,* (*c*) *the same structure as b, but with added noise.* [*Anatomical and physiological terms are written in upper case, and theoretical terms in lower case*].

the input signal from some level defined by the receptor. The box containing the symbol K represents multiplication by a constant, and is usually called gain. Into this are usually lumped factors of proportionality, or dimensions of the system, e.g. the muscle of the iris might contract with so many ergs of force per lumen of light per square cm. of the retina. This proportionality or gain factor is thus a single number which operates multiplicatively on the signal. The effector is simply controlled by this signal and performs its particular function. Fig. 5.2b, then, would be the conceptual informational structure of a simple reflex with feedback.

If this light reflex were entirely of an open loop kind, as in fig. 5.1a, then if the sensitivity of the receptor-retinal system were to change, as it does during dark or light adaptation, or if the counter poise force on the iris muscle were to change as it might if there were some change in the sympathetic system discharge, then this would mean that the proportionality factor (the gain of the system) changed. Thus, for a given amount of light the pupil could be a quite different size depending on these internal changes. Similarly if there were some malfunction in the system its response characteristics would deteriorate, perhaps drastically.

However, because of an apparently minor feature in organization of the components of this reflex pathway, the system's properties are qualitatively different from those just described. The simple arrangement of allowing the response to affect the 'stimulus' that produced it transforms the reflex pathway into a feedback loop, a control system. Clearly the idea of the response feeding back to turn off the stimulus is present in many of Descartes' examples, withdrawing the hand from a fire, blinking etc. Many so-called simple reflexes do indeed have the function of removing something noxious. But the analysis of the reflex, from Descartes to Sherrington and Pavlov, has concentrated on how stimulus produces response, not on the system as having a feedback loop and, therefore, potentially emergent properties. In the pupil system, feedback is clearly present. Reduction in the pupil diameter produced by the light itself reduces the amount of light falling on the retina, so as well as the connection of stimulus to response, there is an informational pathway from response back to stimulus and this is the kind of structure in which we can see novel properties.

In fact many of the properties of such feedback loops are quite general, and can thus be discussed irrespective of their particular physiological embodiment. In fig. 5.2b, this simple feedback loop is described abstractly in informational terms, as having simply an input x, an output y, which is fed back to the comparator, an error signal e which is the difference between x and y, and a gain constant K. Some of the properties of this system can be appreciated qualitatively, i.e. the system operates to minimize the error, so that the output y is closely specified by x. But a quantitative understanding is also possible. One can write down various kinds of equation for the simple feedback loop (Clark Maxwell, 1868, seems to have been the first to do this in a paper whose significance seems not to have been fully appreciated for about seventy years).

The simplest possible analysis, which requires only elementary algebra, is as follows. By definition of the subtractive comparator the error is

$$e = x - y$$

and by definition of the gain, or proportionality factor, the output is,

$$y = Ke.$$

Thus substituting for e, $y = K(x-y)$,

from which
$$y = Kx\text{-}Ky$$
$$y+Ky = Kx$$
$$y(1+K) = Kx$$
and so the output
$$y = \frac{K}{k+1}x$$

Thus the output (y) is shown to be K/1 + K of the input (x) which is the standard or required value. Hence, if the gain (K) is substantially larger than 1, then the fraction K/1 + K approaches K/K, i.e. unity, and thus the ouput is held very close to the prescribed input value. The only difference between the output and desired value is the error: the larger the gain the smaller this error (see fig. 5.2).

Consider now what happens if disturbances, often called noise, affect the system. This can be represented by adding in a noise signal (n) to the pathway, as in fig. 5.2c. As before the error is given by $e = x\text{-}y$

but the output, y, includes the noise, so that
$$y = Ke + n.$$
The output in terms of the input and gain are derived in a similar fashion to that given above
$$Y = K(x\text{-}y)n$$
$$y(1 + K) = Kx + n$$
$$y = \frac{K}{1+K}x + \frac{1}{1+k}n$$

Thus despite disturbances the output y is held to within the distance of the error plus 1/1 + K of the disturbances. That is to say, if the gain is large, the effect of the disturbances is reduced by a factor of approximately K, and the disturbances affect the output very little.

From this kind of organization then arise the properties of regulation, servo-control, and automatic guidance. In principle, with a large gain term the output will closely follow a desired input value, whether this remains steady, as in the physiological system under discussion, or the famous speed control governor used by James Watt for his steam engines. The same principle holds in constantly changing input conditions, as with servo-assisted steering. Also, as Weiner (1958), in his book *Cybernetics* pointed out, these same principles are involved in many biological systems including those described as homeostatic, those involving simple dynamic following of an input signal such as the gamma-efferent servo-system in muscles, and the more complicated tracking and guidance behaviour ranging from eye movement control to some aspects of driving motor cars.

What the control system achieves is relative immunity from disturbance, both from within and without. In a steam locomotive, for instance, if the required speed is specified, something close to that speed will be maintained. If some decrement in the efficiency of the engine occurs, say the fireman forgets to stoke the boiler, then the gain drops, but so long as this gain term is large to start with, it scarcely matters. With a gain of (say) 100, damage to the mechanism or some internal loss of efficiency reducing the gain by half, would only result in an increase of the error from one to two per cent. In the pupil system, too, large changes of efficiency of the internal system have small effects. One is reminded strongly by Lashley's findings of minimal behavioural effect with substantial internal damage. With outside disturbances, too, the feedback loop remains in control. If the steam engine goes up a hill, an increase of load occurs, and the effect of this disturbance is reduced by the size of the gain.

For controllers like automatic guidance systems and autopilots, outside disturbances are not only substantial but rapidly changing. Automatic pilots on small boats, for instance, maintain constant courses with great accuracy despite continual buffeting of the boat by wind and waves. A ground to air guided missile need not be fired accurately. It pursues its quarry with apparent purposefulness and application despite winds tending to divert it, or avoiding action by the aircraft being pursued.

All such devices behave purposefully, keeping constant their output in the face of perturbations if they are regulators, or pursuing an evasive goal if they are guidance systems. Their purposeful behaviour, as Grindley saw, is due in part to their having not one but two inputs, one which is sustained and represents the goal, and the other (which often varies unpredictably) which represents the state of the environment.

The control system of the pupil (described above) has characteristics of regulating the light falling on the retina as has been shown by Stark and Sherman (1957). However, it would be misleading to leave the impression that this is all that there is to be said about the pupil system. The pupil does not serve primarily as does the iris diaphragm in a camera to control the amount of light falling on the photosensitive surface. The analogous function in the eye is served by neural and chemical processes of dark and light adaptation which create changes of sensitivity in the retina. These changes of sensitivity take place across a far greater variation of light intensities than could be coped with by a pupil whose diameter can only vary between 2 and 8 cm.

The pupil is also controlled by the accommodative and convergence systems, so that it constricts as one fixates near objects. As in photography, depth of focus is increased by diminishing the iris diameter. However, visual acuity is also diminished under these conditions, because blur on the retina from diffraction is greater. Pupil size thus depends not only on the lighting conditions; it is also dependent on the distance of the object being viewed, and perhaps also on other characteristics of the object.

MOTIVATIONAL CONTROL SYSTEMS

Homeostatic regulation of behaviour subserving water balance is a further example of a control system, with elements of a type similar to that of light-dependent pupil controller, except that there is a process of integration (in the mathematical sense) in the loop rather than a simple multiplicative gain. Drinking produces a particular rate of intake of water, and thus the volume of the body fluids is increased. Mathematically this transformation of a rate into a volume is represented by the operation of integration (usually depicted as its Laplacian equivalent 1/s in control systems diagrams). This volume is compared with a desired value. When the difference, or deficit reaches a sufficient threshold value, drinking (or water finding behaviour followed by drinking) is generated until the deficit becomes zero (see fig. 5.3). The rate of drinking averaged over time, yields a proportionality or gain constant, and the main difference from the system with a simple purely multiplicative gain term already described, lies in the integration step which necessitates differential equations (or Laplace transforms) rather than simple algebraic ones to express the system properties. Using these, or a computer simulation, it is easy to show again by an apparently slightly change in the organization of the system, i.e. the addition of an integration step (which has the simple physical embodiment of the drinking rate being integrated to contribute to the body fluid volume) that again new properties emerge. In this system, response to a disturbance (e.g. a water deficit acquired through not having drunk for some time, or through body fluid changes consequent

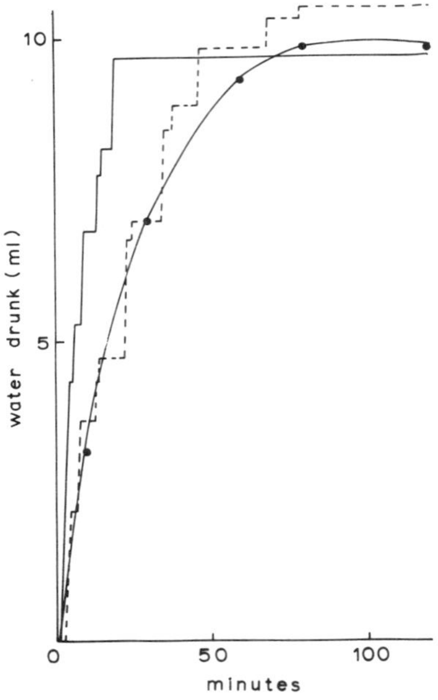

Figure 5.3 Exponential drinking in response to a displacement from body fluid equilibrium. An exponential curve has been drawn through the spots representing the mean amounts drunk by rats following intravenous salt injections in an experiment of Toates and Oatley (1970). The dotted line represents drinking of an individual rat, and the stepwise solid line the drinking simulated by the computer model described by Toates & Oatley.

on eating a dry meal) is gradual and exponential, but now the emergent property is that there is no residual error. A control system with an integration step in it eliminates the error term altogether; instead the gain term determines how fast is the exponential return to the controlled value.

It has been shown in detail (e.g. Toates and Oatley, 1970; Oatley, 1973) how behavioural properties such as purposeful regulation of body water including the control of intake and excretion arise or emerge from a feedback structure. The component processes and their interactions have been simulated by computer and it is the system working as a whole which has the regulatory properties, not any of the component processes.

I shall not recapitulate the evidence and results of that work in detail here, although I will remark that the whole process of simulation, or indeed writing any computer program itself illustrates the emergence of properties from interactions of component parts (i.e. parts of the program). I will simply illustrate the argument with the way in which the structure of feedback loops is not only pressed into service in homeostatic regulation, but with another slight modification also into a source of oscillation which allows timing and complex synchronization of related events.

Feedback control systems, such as that described in figs. 5.2 or 5.3, and the accompanying equations are capable of accomplishing purposeful regulation, but they are also capable of becoming unstable. Typically, this occurs if there are delays in signal transmission in the system. Clearly all physical systems must involve some delays since time is necessarily taken in transmission of a signal, even if the time is very small as in electronic systems. The consequence of such delays is a tendency of the system to oscillate. Consider what happens when someone with a public address system, or a music group with amplifying equipment and microphones, occasionally puts a microphone too close to a loudspeaker, or turns the amplifier gain up too high: the equipment produces an ear-splitting howl. What happens is that the slightest disturbance anywhere in the system is amplified, played through the speaker, and if the microphone is close enough to the speaker, it picks up the sound, which is further amplified and again played through the speaker. This time round the sound (having been amplified) is even louder. It goes round the loop again becoming yet louder until the equipment reaches the limit of its output capacity: and a very loud continuous howl is emitted. The sound can be quieted by either turning down the volume control of the amplifier, or by moving the microphone further from the speaker. Both manoeuvres decrease the gain of the system, one directly as the volume knob controls the gain of the amplifier, the other indirectly as sound is progressively attenuated with increasing distance.

What is happening is that the components, microphone, amplifier and speaker, have been put together in a feedback loop, with the loop being completed by the acoustic transmission of the speaker signal in air to the microphone. If the total gain or net multiplication of the signal round this loop is greater than one, then clearly each time it goes round, the signal grows in size, until the system reaches its maximum output. Only by reducing the net gain of the loop below unity will disturbances fail to increase in this 'vicious circle' fashion.

When howling occurs it takes the form of a simple oscillation and its frequency depends on the loop delay. Thus if the microphone is moved closer to the speaker the travel time of the signal in air is diminished and the tone's pitch becomes higher.

In this case the feedback is an 'accidental' creation, and the emergent property, howling, quite unwanted. It happens, though, that all feedback systems are liable to break into an oscillation in this way, if the gain of the system round the loop is higher than one. Consider the feedback system of fig. 5.2c but with a delay in the feeback path. If a tiny random perturbation occurs, it will be fed back to the comparator, and a compensatory counteraction of larger size initiated. If the disturbance and counterthrust are simultaneous, then the properties of regulation occur as shown in the equations given. If, however, there is any delay in the loop, the counterthrust will be a little too late to counteract the disturbance. Instead it will act as a new disturbance in the opposite direction to the original, and by now larger by a factor equivalent to the gain of the loop. This new disturbance again travels round. Again, the comparator produces an error of opposite sign, which is again multiplied and arrives too late to act as a compensation.

Just as in the case of the microphone and speaker the disturbance grows. Each passage round the loop is half a cycle of an oscillation, since each passage produces an amplified signal in the opposite direction to the last. The period of the oscillation which builds up is, by the same token, twice the time taken to traverse the loop.

Since (as shown above) in practical regulators the gain must be high to produce the properties of regulation, and since in all physical systems the signal must take time to travel round the loop (i.e. it is delayed), the incipient break into unstable oscillation seems to contradict the possibility of making any practical regulator. However, there is a way out of the difficulty. The unstable oscillation builds up at only one frequency (the reciprocal of twice the loop delay), and so if the gain of the system could be made less than one for that frequency, then the system would be able to regulate perfectly well for signals changing more slowly. This is the type of solution sought by engineers who design control systems. It is also the arrangement that exists in biological regulators.

Of course, with this solution, if the gain of the whole system were to rise for some reason, the gain at the unstable oscillation frequency might exceed unity, and an unstable oscillation break out, even in usually stable systems. Such an outcome can be achieved in the pupil control system discussed above and studied by Stark and Sherman (1957). The gain of the loop can be artificially increased by shining a thin beam of light on the edge of the pupil. This increases the gain because now a small movement of the pupil produces a much larger change of light intensity on the retina than in the normal course of events. The result is that the pupil goes into a violent oscillation (called by opthalmologists induced puillary hippus, a largely incomprehensible state before this kind of analysis). The oscillation has a period which is twice the reaction time of the pupil to a light stimulus. Normally in its regulatory mode the gain of the system at this unstable frequency is less than one, and the pupil is controlled by the light input.

The oscillation which thus develops in feedback systems is an emergent property, arising because of a particular arrangement of parts, but in no sense a property of, or contained as an essence in, any particular part. In the case of regulatory control systems including biological systems, this behaviour is prevented by making the gain at the oscillation frequency small. The diminution in gain as a function of frequency of oscillation, or rate of change of the input events, is a further emergent property. I have shown elsewhere (Oatley and Toates, 1971) both that this property is exhibited by a typical biological homeostat, the drinking control system, and how it emerges from the control structure which contains an integration step in its forward pathway (though the property is not contained in the integration step).

A precise characterization of how the gain of a simple control system decreases with increasing frequency requires an excursion into calculus which seems a bit inappropriate here. Rather I will try to give some intuitions about how the property emerges. The system is one in which there are rates (i.e. rates of drinking and excretion) which are proportional to volumes (i.e. of body fluids). Such systems in which a rate is proportional to an integral are known as first order systems, and can be described by first order differential equations. The gain term, K, now describes the rate of integration. I said above that this term determined the rate of exponential response to a sudden input. For a high gain the response is swift, and for a low gain it is more gradual. It follows that with input signals that are changing (e.g. an oscillation which changes direction in an alternating fashion), the system will be able to 'keep up' with the oscillation at low frequencies, i.e. it will be able to follow a slowly oscillating waveform almost to the extent of the waveform's total upwards and downwards swings. For a faster oscillation, however, the total apparent gain of the whole loop will be lower, because, as the input waveform changes direction, the output will not be at its maximum excursion, and will start to change direction before reaching the maximum excursion. The higher the frequency, the lower the amplitude of the output oscillation, as the rate limitation makes the system less and less able to follow the rapid input alternations with maximum amplitude.

A mechanical analogy (or example) of a first order system's rate limitation is the spring and shock absorber suspension of a car. In a spring the force is proportional to the spring's extension or compression. In a shock absorber, the force is proportional to the rate of change of displacement. This relationship of these two components is formally similar to the relationship of rate being proportional to volume described above, i.e. one of the terms is an integral with respect to the other. Moreover, the shock absorber cannot be compressed or extended instantaneously; it takes time to move it. If the car travels along low frequency undulations, the system transmits them to their full amplitude. The rate limitation of the shock absorbers is small in comparison with the rate of undulation. For higher frequency conditions, the transmitted oscillations are diminished or damped. It is precisely the function of the shock absorbers in conjunction with the springs, arranged carefully within the structure of the car's suspension system, to provide the kind of rate limitation which ensures that rapidly changing inputs from the road (such as might occur if the car ran over a brick followed by a pothole) are not transmitted to the chassis at full amplitude.

In the homeostat, then, the tendency of the control structure to create oscillations has been damped, in a manner analogous to the way the spring and shock absorber system provides damping in a car. But as a further example of the inventiveness of biological systems, there is another whole set of applications in which the tendency of the control loop to oscillate has been selected and put to use, in biological rhythms. Here the oscillation does build up, but it is neither damped out nor allowed to become unstable and incapacitate the system. Instead its amplitude is limited and the oscillation is the system's stable state.

All that is necessary for this limitation of the range of oscillation is that the system be non-linear in a particular way. In other words, instead of the gain staying fixed throughout the range of operation of the system, the effective gain becomes small as the amplitude of the signal becomes large. Thus, the extent of the oscillatory swing of the signal is limited. This condition is easily accomplished if the feedback, rather than being a process allied to the mathematical operation of subtraction as in fig. 5.2 and the accompanying equations, is instead an inhibitory process allied to the operation of division.

Such inhibition turns out to be the usual form in biochemical control systems, where, for instance, in protein synthesis a product of a chain of reactions feeds back to inhibit a gene site, or where a product of a chain of enzyme reactions feeds back to inhibit one of the earlier enzyme steps. In each case the rate of the forward reaction is proportional to the amount of the inhibitor, a process like division.

Neural inhibition, too, can be a non-linear process, so that here also the same kind of effect can occur. In this context Cowan (e.g. 1972) has derived equations for non-linear neural oscillations, e.g. of reciprocal inhibition by cortical and thalamic neurones. Such circuits, he argues, are responsible for the oscillatory form of E.E.G. patterns. He further argues that much of the brain's electrical activity, as well as its information processing capacity, can be thought of as being based on the activity of populations of these non-linear oscillators.

I will not pursue that argument here. Rather I wish to consider how such simple biochemical or neural oscillators have properties which emerge, and make them suitable for the workings of biological clocks.

In another article (Oatley, 1974) I have described in detail how a series of standard biochemical reactions can form a feedback loop. Recapitulating this description we can start with a standard equation for enzyme reaction. It is derived from the Michaelis-Menton equation, but there is also a term to represent an inhibitor.

$$\frac{du}{dt} = \frac{L}{A + Bz} - Ku.$$

Here du is the rate of formation of the substance u. It depends on constants L, A and B, and the rate is diminished by the presence of the inhibitor substance z. (The inhibition is represented as a division; z appears in the denominator of the equation.) Ku represents the transport of u away from the reaction at a rate K. Now in biochemical systems there are typically several other processes, each taking a certain amount of time (equivalent to exponential lags), and these can be designated as processes successively producing substances v, w, x, y and z. The substance z, as I said, is, however, the inhibitor of the first process, described by the above equation. The whole chain of processes thus constitutes a feedback loop, and its output is a so-called non-linear oscillation. It is non-linear in the sense that the equation above is a non-linear differential equation; the division or inhibition by z varies the effective gain of the process throughout its cycle and the oscillation

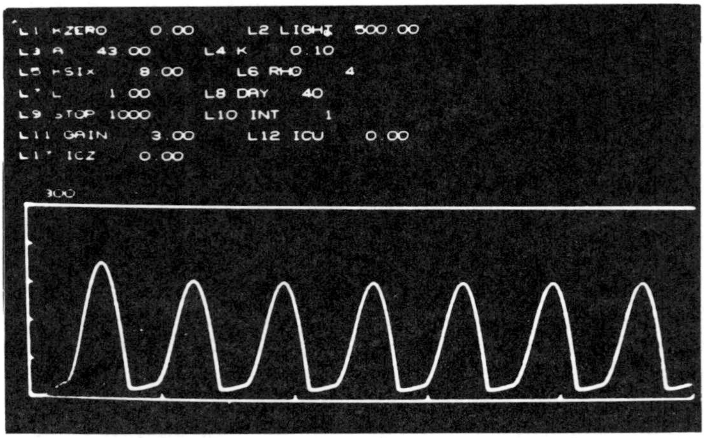

Figure 5.4 Photograph of a non-linear oscillation seen on a computer visual display. It is the output of a simulation program (described by Oatley, 1974), solving an equation of the kind described above; numbers in the top half of the picture are parameter values.

produced is non-sinusoidal. The waveshape of this particular process as seen from a computer simulation is illustrated in fig. 5.4

Functions of biological rhythms have been discussed at length elsewhere (e.g. Oatley and Goodwin, 1971; Oatley, 1974, 1975), but basically rhythms can be thought of as processes which allow animals to synchronize their activities with the outer environment, e.g. the sleep rhythm with the pattern of night and day, and also to synchronize related internal processes with each other; e.g. maintaining the correct timing sequences in a series of psychological, neural, developmental, or biochemical events.

The equation described above merely expresses rates of reaction for simple biochemical processes. In one sense the processes are just enzyme reactions. But in another sense the system of reactions is not just a regulated factory for making a few chemicals. It is, for instance, a hormonal or neurochemical clock, and properties emerge from the process which fit it for that function.

The alternating pattern of the oscillation as a biological clock is, amongst other things, an internal representation of the alternating pattern of light and darkness. It is by such representations or models of the rotation of the earth that neural processes such as sleep are controlled, not by direct observation of the outside environment. We do not feel sleepy simply when someone switches out the light. Rather sleepiness is induced primarily by an internal process, which has the same rhythm as the environmental cycle of night and day and keeps in time with that environmental state.

The kind of non-linear oscillator described above as arising simply from a feedback loop of biochemical processes, as well as generating a suitable cycle to act as a clock, has this additional emergent property of enabling the internal clock to keep in time, or synchronize itself on the external lighting cycle. All non-linear oscillators, as it happens, have this capacity for entrainment. This means that if a periodic event, at a frequency near the natural frequency of the non-linear oscillator, can in any way affect it, then the oscillator tends to become synchronized with the external frequency source. The process can be seen in the mutual entrainment of two artificial clocks placed close together (Huygens, 1665).

Entrainment occurs because the underlying process is

non-linear: both the rate and sensitivity of the process to outside effects varies over the cycle. An external event occurring at the most sensitive part of the cycle may speed up the process slightly. This will have the effect of increasing the frequency, and if the external event is also periodic and at, say, a slightly higher frequency, the oscillator will move in frequency and phase until a state is reached where the external event is adding just enough energy to keep the oscillator in time with it. Were the non-linear cycle to move forward any more, then the external events would start to fall in a less sensitive part of the cycle. Thus an entrained equilibrium can occur.

Circadian clocks mostly entrain on the light-dark pattern of the environment. With the kind of oscillator described above, this merely requires that some reaction in the sequence be light-sensitive, like, for instance, the reaction in the production of melatonin which is catalysed by the enzyme hydroxyindole-o-methyl transferase. Alternatively, some neuro-chemical process deriving from the visual system might affect one of the stages of the oscillator and thus provide the entrainment signal.

Simulation of these biological clock mechanisms by computer has shown that this entrainment property emerges directly from the structure discussed above, and entrainment on different frequencies, and re-entrainment following a phase reversal occurs (see e.g. Oatley, 1975).

Properties of the feedback loop, control, regulation and entrainable oscillation clearly emerge as properties of the organization of processes in a feedback loop not the individual processes themselves. Indeed, the properties are independent of whether the underlying process is electrical, biochemical, mechanical or neural. It is the organization of connections among components in a particular fashion in a loop which gives rise to regulatory and oscillatory properties. Furthermore, the fact that properties do emerge from even simply interacting processes makes the reductionistic identification of behaviour with parts of a highly interconnected interactive brain, very suspect.

The feedback structure is non-reflexlike in that properties like purposefulness emerge from it. Moreover, it defies the usual breakdown of behaviour into isolation of stimulus and response, and identification of their neural (or conceptual) connection. It directs our attention to investigating principles of complex informational interactions, not just the nuts and bolts of a system.

As mentioned early in the chapter, for Lashley too the closed loop structure held a fascination, and he repeatedly drew attention to the discovery by Lorente de No (1933) of recurrent neural networks. Perhaps the attraction was that such arrangements represented a type of neural organization which one could see under the microscope, and which was evidently unreflexlike. In other words, here was a new organization from which new properties might emerge. And this organization was pressed into service not only as an explanation for sustained motivational states, but for the formation of dynamic patterns of neural organization. 'An excited cell transmits impulses to adjacent cells, and the excitation may be returned from various distances, through one or a thousand links. Since the activation or inhibition of a cell is dependent upon the number and frequency of the impulses transmitted to it, it is obvious that a system so organized will have its own inherent patterns of response.' (1949) It seems that in these continuously active, yet organized patterns, 'neural schemata' as Lashley called them, that Lashley hoped to find principles underlying the emergent properties of mind. In 1942, indeed, he had even made an attempt at explaining how the intrinsically dynamic, yet stable patterns of activity somewhat like waves, on the surface of a liquid (cf. the oscillations described above). However, since the cortex is not homogeneous like a liquid there will be a greater organization of these patterns from the neural structure itself. 'Spatially distributed impulses reaching the cortex from the retina ... will give rise to a ... characteristic pattern of standing waves reduplicated throughout the extent of the functional area.'

One can sense that Lashley armed with the notion of the dynamically active cortex, with intrinsic patterns of oscillatory activity, and his metaphor of waves with patterns of resonance, diffraction, interference and so on, is feeling for a solution to all the problems of stimulus and motor equivalence, mass action, coherently structured behaviour and so forth, that he had spent a lifetime grappling with. Yet the attempt does not quite succeed. Lashley seems to have seen potential emergence of important properties in the structure of recurrent neural paths, yet he could not spell this out. In most of his writings he stressed the importance of meaning. Yet basically his patterns of waves and diffraction patterns and so on are just a more complex, wholistic expression of the notion that the problem of understanding behaviour is to understand how stimulus is connected to response. 'The transition from the visual perceptual to the motor level thus appears to be, primitively, the translation of one system of space co-ordinates into another' (1942). Thus, Lashley sees the visual system primarily concerned with spatial co-ordinates. He then sees some mediating process, perhaps analogous to wave phenomena which translates these co-ordinates into the terms of the motor system by modifying its pattern of postural organization. His model makes an attempt at explaining stimulus equivalence, mass action and motor equivalence. It is still recognizably a stimulus-response formulation.

One of the properties one hopes would emerge from some adequate analogy for the brain is meaning, and this is just what Lashley's or anyone else's stimulus response formulation lacks.

Let me by returning to the structure of the biological clock suggest an alternative, a representation within which one can speak of meaning, and which may also be able to address the problems of mass action and so on.

Biological clocks, perhaps better than any other well understood example, illustrate a fundamental pattern of interaction with the environment, the structure of which is as follows. First, there is the outside world, which is rich, complex and diverse. Secondly, there is within an organism adapted to that environment an internal model of some aspect or aspects of that environment. These aspects are of functional relevance or importance to the life of the organism in that environment. Thirdly, there are the interactions of the organism and its model with the environment. Typically these interactions are in two directions: the ways in which the environment or its 'relevant' aspects affect the internal model, and the ways in which the organism acts on the environment to change that environment, or at least to change its relationship to the environment, which amounts to the same thing as far as the organism is concerned.

In the specific case of biological clocks, the relevant aspect embodied in the model is primarily the alternation of light and darkness, which has significance for sleeping and activity amongst other things. (There are also further aspects related, for instance, to navigation in species with particular kinds of adaptation to their world.) The way the internal model works is by exhibiting a structure and a behaviour which can model or mirror particular aspects: it is a representation, a schema which contains knowledge of certain characteristics of the world (e.g. of the alternation of light and darkness). The knowledge is, however, abstracted in that it represents only a very partial analysis of the environment. It is not neutral in the sense that knowledge in an encyclopedia typically is. There knowledge is neutral in that an attempt has been made not to presuppose the uses to which the knowledge may be put. In the biological schema a quite different situation obtains. The knowledge is both committed (or biased) and embedded in a procedure or process which includes what the organism is to do about the world, and what it might infer about selected aspects of the world. Thus on the 'input' side the biological clock's relationship with the environment is characterized by a sensitivity to entrainment by the external lighting cycle and on the 'output' side by initiation or creation of both behaviour and physiological processes appropriate to light or darkness (e.g. sleep, the increased secretion of growth hormone etc.).

In this structure we can if we wish see the elements of the reflex. The entraining effect of light could be seen as a stimulus, the biological clock as a connection, sleep as a response. But these terms impoverish the phenomena. They express neither emergent properties nor meaning. Whereas the analysis in terms of schemata (and their emergent properties) carries forward an understanding of the meaningful relationships of organisms with their worlds. The stimulus-connection-response notion tends to dismiss meaning. With the idea of schemata we can give some account of phenomena ranging from the very simplest examples in this chapter of purposeful regulation by means of an internally symbolized goal or desired state in a control system, or activities meaningfully structured in time, to some of the more complex human activities, such as the deployment of metaphor in art, or theory in science. In these latter instances, too, the structure is of an internal representation being put in relation to some aspect of the world, to understand it, to give it meaning, or to come to terms with it, or to do something about it.

Consider the following, from Clowes (1973).

> Metaphors, representations, theories, don't (or shouldn't) claim to be the thing they explain; only devices to add insight into what they explain ... In Bartlett's phrase 'the immediately present stands for something not immediately present'. How does 'stand for' work? How is it possible that A can stand for B? Why connect up A (here) to B (not present)? So that you can mobilize inferences bound to B.

In this biological clock, lighting cycles of the present environment are made to 'stand for' the non-linear oscillation – why? In order to mobilize the inferences bound to and the procedures embedded in the clock, e.g. to promote sleeping or waking appropriately. The activity here is not available to conscious introspection to be sure, but the structure of internal representation is present. (I would like to note here that 'stand for' in Bartlett's phrase is the environment 'standing for' the schema, but the reverse usage, of the schema 'standing for' the environment seems equally good.) Let me add that it is this structure of representation within, of aspects of the world without, that I wish to argue makes a lot more sense of psychology and neurophysiology than the stimulus-connections-response formulation.

In the next chapter I will explore some of the further 'meaningful' properties of representations. Then in the subsequent two chapters I will give an analysis of perception in these terms, and an account of how some of Lashley's problems of 'stimulus and response equivalence' and mass action are informed by this analysis.

6 *Representations and schemata*

In understanding emergent properties of biological systems, we find that symbolic processes emerge from inter-relations of biochemical and neural events. Thus a key to how a simple homeostatic control system works is the idea that the desired level, set point or whatever, is really an internal representation of an aspect of the outside world. Purposefulness implies a desired state of the environment, which could exist in the future, but does not exist in the present. In order to avoid absurdities such as having future events causing present events, purposefulness must be accomplished using some symbolic representation of the environment, e.g. a representation of a desired state or goal.

It is the structure of a homeostatic feedback system which gives the set point, or desired or reference level this role. This internal representation of a possible state of some aspect of the environment is needed amongst other things for comparisons with that aspect of the current environment, to produce an error signal and thus a steering action towards the goal.

The set point and comparator system may, as in the case of one of these structures in the thirst system, be physiologically speaking a non-adapting receptor. But the inter-relations and interactions it has with other parts of the system confer upon it an emergent informational role. Thus, the finding that thirst osmoreceptors do not adapt (e.g. Fitzsimons, 1963) is a physiological interpretation. It can also be thought of in informational terms as a statement that the current osmotic concentration of the body fluid is compared with a fixed value, representing a relatively invariable desired state.

As Grindley (1927) pointed out, it is in general upon such arrangements of an internal innervation specifying a goal and input from the outside world that purposive behaviour can be built.

As it turns out, the homeostat has only limited value in the generation of behaviour. It copes with deficits, but it cannot predict them or take avoiding action. Anticipation requires different and more powerful representations of the environment, and a simple case is provided by circadian oscillators which act as models of the rotation of the earth, and the alternation of night and day.

The advantages of organizing behaviour around a model of the rotation of the earth, rather than simply around direct observations of the ambient lighting are that direct observations cannot always be made (e.g. if one is down a dark hole), predictions can be made, so that one can, for instance, anticipate the dawn. Furthermore, with the entrainment phenomena of biological clocks, complex timing relationships can be supported between related processes.

Internal representations (which themselves are symbolic systems with properties that emerge as a result of the interactions of their components) are thus fundamental to even rather simple kinds of behaviour. Reflex theories may allow us to overlook the importance of internal symbolic processes, but feedback structures do not.

In these almost foolishly simple examples it is possible to glimpse something of the alternative of seeing behaviour not simply as reacting to stimulus patterns from the outside world, but of using internal models of that outside world to interact purposefully, and appropriately with it.

It is clear that the representations we have of our world, its layout in space, the potentialities of various objects in it, the plans we can make for some course of action, are all much more complex than the limited and special purpose representations within control systems. But it may be that the richness of the possible representations an animal or person might have comes close to what we mean by intelligence.

As an illustration of apparently unintelligent behaviour, which is nevertheless evidently effective in maintaining the species, Lashley (1949) cites the behaviour of the sooty tern (which he studied in 1915). The nesting tern will attack any birds intruding into her territory, and defend her chicks if they are attacked by neighbours. However, if she has rescued a chick from such an attack she will herself immediately run towards the chick, and attack it if it runs away. But it runs towards her, and nestles under her breast. She responds to this with a protective hovering reaction. Finding herself away from the nest she may then get up and walk back towards the nest, but now if the chick is left behind she will turn and move towards it again, and so on. In time both mother and chick get back to the nest. The behaviour of the mother tern here is evidently under the immediate control of a rather small number of aspects of the situation. It appears absurd because there are other aspects, other relationships in the situation which she does not seem to take into account, and a human observer can.

Evidently the mother tern's representation of the problem of getting the chick back to the nest (if it is reasonable to talk about her having a representation rather than a set of stimulus response relations) is an impoverished one. If the mother-chick pair understood more about the consequences of actions and the inter-relationship between them, they might behave more 'sensibly', more appropriately.

Similar behaviour which was effective in securing a result, but which could be labelled 'unintelligent', is exhibited by cortical lesioned rats solving puzzle box problems. Lashley (1949) argued that these lesions in rats, though not necessarily reducing the animals' ability to perform a task, reduces the complexity of the behaviour, and the animals' insight into the nature of the problem they are solving. Thus, Lashley describes the solution of a double latch box task. To open the box and reach food, a rat had first to press a lever then step on a platform to open the door. A normal rat at first operates the latch by climbing on it or stepping on it by accident. After a few trials his behaviour changes. He may then seize the lever with his teeth and operate it, and then make a quick turn and thrust down with his forefeet on the platform which releases the door. The rat's movements become economically directed to those features of the situation that are effective in operating the latches. Rats with large cortical lesions can learn the task in about the same number of trials as normal rats, but their behaviour seems simplified. One rat with 40 per cent of his cortex missing, for instance, first opened the door by scrambling over the latch and then falling off backwards onto the platform. He continued to use this same rather inelegant procedure throughout training. He was able to reach food as quickly as a normal animal, but as Lashley remarks 'His reactions were organized at a simpler level, as associated movements without insight into the significance of the latches.'

There is a difficulty here: as is characteristic when discussing the effects of lesions, the behaviour of the operated rat could be described as less complex than normal, and Lashley used this (one suspects) as an anecdotal illustration to expound his view of the nature of intelligence. It is not clear that anyone since Lashley has advanced more plausible views, but a critic could equally well describe the behaviour of the lesioned rat in the latch box in quite other terms than simplification and lack of insight. Perhaps the lesion made the animal less active, so that fewer spontaneous variaitons of his original successful response were produced, and thus the variations which might be described as more economical or insightful solutions were not available for reinforcement. It is not that Lashley's conclusion is wrong; simply that the data he presents do not make it universally convincing. It is precisely from this kind of issue that there grows the whole line of research into the making of experimental brain lesions and trying to define the exact way in which behaviour is altered by them.

What might be more apposite would be to follow the other strand of Lashley's thought; to enquire what representations are, what kinds of representations animals and people have of their environments, what the psychology of such representations might be and what their characteristics are.

Representations and symbols are made possible because different physical objects have common properties or aspects. Thus, a resistor and capacitor in an electrical network can represent mechanical components; the shock absorber and spring in a car's suspension (or indeed the rate-volume relationship between drinking and body fluids discussed in the previous chapter). Both resistor and shock absorber dissipate energy, while both capacitor and spring store it. For all components the characteristics are fairly constant over a wide range. The electrical, mechanical and body fluid systems can, moreover, be represented in yet another symbolic description, a differential equation. A first order linear equation not only describes the systems well; it abstracts what they hold in common. Moreover, the electrical network of capacitor and resistor can also be called an analogue computer and used to solve differential equations.

Digital computers can be representational too. Their components signal simply two states, but these can be put into correspondence with any disjunction, yes or no, one or zero, possessing some property or lacking it, so that concatenation of such symbolic elements makes the computer universal, capable of simulating or representing almost anything that one can specify exactly.

It is because of the possibility of symbolic representation that brains and minds exist. Although all kinds of things can represent each other, brains and computers seem both to have evolved specifically to mobilize and make use of this representational aspect. And if brains principally have this aspect and function, one of the threads of argument in this book is that we should approach them accordingly. The idea has, however, all kinds of apparently unfortunate consequences for brain research. Because representational properties emerge from interacting structures the paradigmatic scientific technique of isolating a particular component to study it may be less useful than it seems. Conversely because it is often possible to represent the informational properties of a process in a language (such as a computer program) which is free of the implications of any particular embodiment in neurones, or electronics or cogwheels, developments in understanding system properties offer no particular biological specification of the underlying process. Indeed the relationships between underlying processes and symbolic properties can remain very obscure. But if the brain is a symbolic representational device, then these are consequences which brain research must confront.

What then is known of representational processes in general, and those of the human brain in particular? One of the principal features of a representation of an environment or a problem is that a particular representation is more or less adequate for a particular purpose. Any given representation is not typically equally good for a variety of purposes. In a guide book, for instance, a map may be a good representation for telling one how to get to some place. But something quite different involving words or pictures is necessary to tell one whether it might be worth going there.

This specificity of representation to particular tasks can be demonstrated both informally and formally. As an example of the informal type of illustration, consider the following two problems.

Problem 1 (Adapted from Duncker, 1945) A man sets off with his rucksack and tent to climb a mountain. He leaves a small village in the valley at 8.00 a.m. and climbs upwards along a well marked narrow track, stopping from time to time to admire the view or to have something to eat or drink. He arrives at the top at about 5.00 p.m. and makes camp. The next day after breakfast he sets off down the mountain starting again at 8.00 a.m., and following exactly the same track. But though he again makes short stops, he completes the journey down somewhat more quickly than the journey up and arrives at his starting place at 3.00 p.m. The question is 'Is there any position on the mountain track that the man reached at exactly the same time of day on his downward journey as he did on the ascent?'

To start with this seems like a rather muddling question. One juggles with times, and notions of the top, bottom and middle of the mountain. Perhaps we think of representations like algebra, or graphs. But thinking of the man walking up on one day and down on the next, we probably come to no particular conclusion; except perhaps that he probably did pass the same place at the same time, otherwise the problem would not have been put.

If, however, the problem is transformed; giving it a new representation not of one man on two successive days, but of two men on the same day, leaving and arriving at the times specified, then the muddle disappears. One man starts from the top, the other starts at the same time from the bottom. Do they reach the same place at the same instant? Of course they do, because they must pass each other. Within this representation the problem and its solution become clear and unequivocal. If one can cast it into a form within which we can reason effectively, the problem becomes easy.

Problem 2 Imagine a square of paper 8 inches by 8 inches. Now imagine that you cut out a one inch square from each of two diametrically opposite corners (see fig. 6.1). The problem

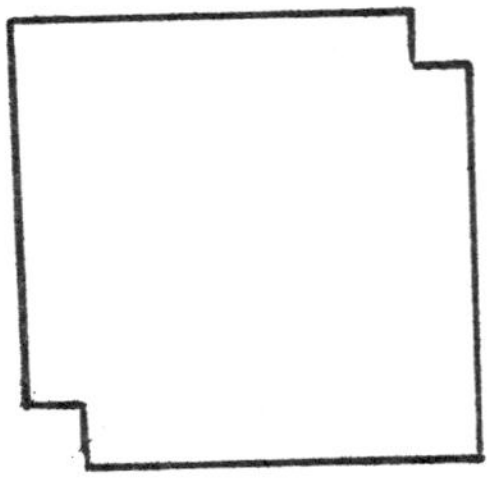

Figure 6.1 Square with diagonally opposite corners cut out.

is 'Is it possible to cover the remaining area completely with no overlap and no pieces sticking out, with little rectangles of card that are each two inches by one inch?' Now this is a problem which most people applying their ordinary representations find impossibly difficult. One might mentally fill in the bottom row, starting at the side with the missing corner, and put in three rectangles horizontally, and then one vertical one at the end. One might repeat this pattern, zigzagging up to the top. Doing it this way (if we can hold this kind of process in our imagination, or if we use a piece of paper) we find that we cannot cover all the squares. But we are still confused as to whether perhaps some other arrangement would do it.

There is, however, another representation or schema for this problem which immediately makes it easier. If the original 8 × 8 square were a chess board, then the two corner pieces that would have been removed would either have been both black or both white. On the other hand, any 2 × 1 piece of card must cover one black and one white square, and therefore the answer is that no arrangement of these 2 × 1 pieces of card could conceivably cover the whole board, because there is either going to be two white squares or two black squares left at the end, and these cannot be horizontally or vertically adjacent.

Thus again with one representation of the problem it seems impossibly difficult, with another it becomes feasible. There are many such puzzles, and there are several distinguished contributions to the problem of how people can improve their problem solving by understanding better the issue of task representation (e.g. Wertheimer, *Productive Thinking*, 1961 and Polya, *How to Solve It*, 1945).

One apposite and revealing analysis of the importance of appropriate representational structures for a particular task has been in computational problem solving and game playing. There are many examples, but the following is simple and quite instructive. It concerns the games of noughts and crosses (tic-tac-toe in America).

Suppose you wanted to write a computer program to play noughts and crosses, one of the basic problems is 'How do you represent the playing space in the best way to allow your program to win or draw?' Clearly, noughts and crosses is a relatively simple game for people, and a competent player need never lose: two competent players always draw. But what kind of representation in the mind or a program will facilitate appropriate strategies?

Clearly there has to be some means for representing each of the nine positions, some means for denoting whether they contain a nought or a cross, or are empty. Ideally also this representation should make it easy for the program to identify how to play to make a line, or avoid the opponent doing so.

Perhaps the first way one might think of would be to set up nine cells labelled 1 to 9 in sequence, and fill them with symbols, say 0 for nought, 1 for cross, and 2 for empty. However, this scheme, though it is sufficient to identify all possible states and conditions of the game, is extremely clumsy. For instance, the essence of the game is to make lines of three markers across, downwards or diagonally. Yet there is nothing simple about the labels 1 to 9 to signify that (say), square number 2 is in a line with square 5 (see fig. 6.2a). One might do better by labelling the cells 1,1; 1,2; 1,3; 2,1 etc as in fig. 6.2b. Now it is easy to test whether, for instance, two noughts or two crosses are in the same row or column, such that the next move would be a potential win. One simply has to check whether either the first or the second of the cell-identifying digits is the same. This then is a representation in which the idea of rows and columns is contained as well as the idea of adjacency and distance in a row or column.

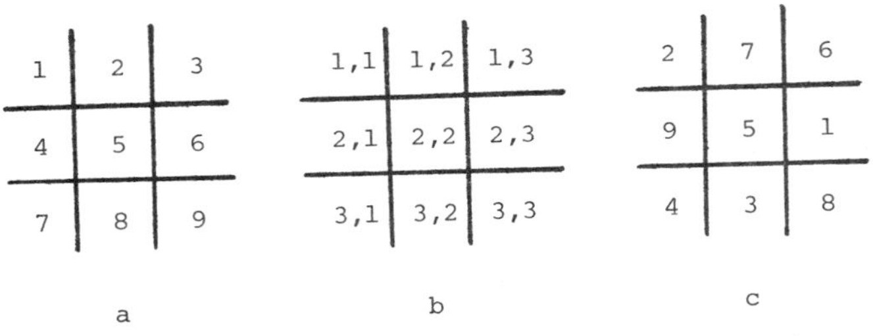

Figure 6.2 Representations for noughts and crosses (see text).

However, the diagonals are still difficult to handle under this scheme. Certainly they require different treatment from rows and columns, which is a nuisance. A rather surprising representation which avoids that difficulty is to use the idea of the magic number square, see fig. 6.2c. Here digits 1 to 9 are again used, but in such a fashion that the sum of digits in any row, column or diagonal, is 15. Now with this representation the game becomes that of placing the symbols in such a way as to occupy any three cells whose number-labels sum to 15.

Apparently then this representation fits the task of playing the game quite well. However, it is still not very good. A program based on the magic number square and with the basic strategy of placing its token on the third of any three cells whose number-labels sum to 15, if the first two are occupied both by noughts or both by crosses, will hold its own against a fairly naive player but will lose to anyone using a forcing move. Such a move would be made by 'noughts' in the following game.

1 Nought in top right corner.
Cross in centre.
2 Nought in bottom left corner
(opposite corner of a diagonal).

'Noughts' have now applied a forcing pattern. Although a win for 'noughts' is not inevitable from this move; unless 'crosses' make the next move correctly, they will lose. If, for instance, they continue:

Cross in bottom right corner

there may follow

3 Nought in top left corner.

Now there are two lines which will potentially win for 'noughts', see fig. 6.3, whereas 'crosses' can only block one of these on the next move. The trap would be avoided at 'crosses' move 2 by playing in the centre position of any side.

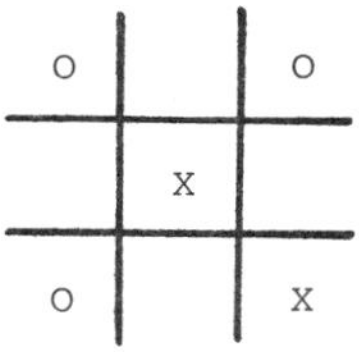

Figure 6.3 A forcing pattern in noughts and crosses.

There is nothing in the magic number square representation as such which would either make it easy to produce or counter the strategies of forcing moves. Thus either some addition to or improvement of the representational structure is again required.

A further step might, therefore, be to try and describe the playing space in such a way as to make forcing strategies easy to operate. As described above, this would need to take advantage of the symmetry of the board, and the various strategic positions, i.e. the centre, opposite corners of a diagonal etc. At this stage the representation would start (perhaps) to come a bit closer to the one that people use.

Even in this short sequence, in a rather childish game, one can begin to see the importance of having the good representations, and that any given representation is going to be more or less fit for a specific job. Thus it is most important in psychology and brain research to understand what actual behavioural and ecological purposes are served by particular mental processes. Without knowing the purposes or aims of a brain mechanism or a piece of behaviour it is difficult to see how we are likely to get on the right lines towards understanding it. If one thinks of almost any simple machine, e.g. a lawn mower, bicycle pump, or a fountain pen, its particular design and workings are intimately part of what it has to do. If we know what it does, it is often not too difficult to see what role various parts have, why the parts are arranged in the way they are, and how the whole things works. If we had no idea (or theory) of what even the simplest machine did, its workings could remain very mysterious.

One of the problems with creating new species of animal, by making brain lesions in existing species, is that rather than simplifying the behavioural repertoire, the lesion could be thought of as creating a new problem of being able to understand yet another kind of animal. Furthermore, this new animal is less likely to be well adapted to any environment. Thus understanding its behaviour might be made more, not less, difficult, because of the absence of help we can get from our ideas of the function of the behaviour.

Schemata then are representations of knowledge more or less well fitted (so far as we can understand) to particular tasks. There are varieties of representations for any given task or arrangement of the environment, and perhaps in evolution, in learning and in cultural development what goes on is the acquisition of more appropriate, more powerful schemata.

Hughlings Jackson spoke of representations in the brain (see chapter 4) and subsequently another neurologist, Head (1920), talked of schemata as indeed did Lashley (see chapter 5). But one of the best accounts is given by Bartlett (1932) in his analyses of successive rememberings of meaningful stories.

Bartlett used a method of asking English subjects to read through twice a translation of a folk story from another culture (e.g. in the example below an American Indian folk tale), and then write it out as exactly as possible on a number of occasions days and weeks, and in a few cases years, after the initial readings. One story used was as follows:

THE WAR OF THE GHOSTS

One night two young men from Egulac went down to the river to hunt seals, and while they were there it became foggy and calm. They heard war-cries and they thought: 'Maybe this is a war party'. They escaped to the shore, and hid behind a log. Now canoes came up, and they heard the noise of paddles, and saw one canoe coming up to them. There were five men in the canoe, and they said:

'What do you think? We wish to take you along. We are going up the river to make war on the people.'

One of the young men said: 'I have no arrows.'

'Arrows are in the canoe', they said.

'I will not go along. I might be killed. My relatives do not know where I have gone. But you', he said, turning to the other, 'may go with them.'

So one of the young men went, but the other returned home.

And the warriors went on up the river to a town on the other side of Kalama. The people came down to the water, and they began to fight, and many were killed. But presently the young man heard one of the warriors say: 'Quick, let us go home: that Indian has been hit.' Now he thought: 'Oh, they are ghosts.' He did not feel sick, but they said he had been shot.

So the canoes went back to Egulac, and the young man went ashore to his house, and made a fire. And he told everybody and said: 'Behold I accompanied the ghosts, and we went to fight. Many of our fellows were killed, and many of those who attacked us were killed. They said I was hit, and I did not feel sick.'

He told it all, and then he became quiet. When the sun rose he fell down. Something black came out of his mouth. His face became contorted. The people jumped up and cried.

He was dead.

In general, as might be expected, one major change that takes place on reproduction is a shortening of the original length. But this is not due simply to omission of material. Rather the person making the reproduction is actively contributing something. Here, for instance, is the first part of one of Bartlett's subjects' reproductions after an interval of 20 hours.

'Two men from Edulac went fishing. While thus occupied by the river they heard a noise in the distance.

"It sounded like a cry", said one, and presently there appeared some men in canoes who invited them to join the party on their adventure. One of the young men refused to go on the grounds of family ties, but the other offered to go.'

The striking thing about this is the replacement of what Bartlett calls the inconsequential tone of the original story by modern phraseology, somewhat in the style of a rather bad newspaper, e.g. 'refused to go on the grounds of family ties', and later in this subject's reproduction 'The enemy came rushing upon them, and some sharp fighting ensued' etc.

Also in this subject's efforts the issue of the ghosts was transformed from the young man accompanying ghosts to the battle in the original to the idea that only the enemy were ghosts: i.e. in this subject's reproduction: 'Presently someone was injured, and the cry was raised that the enemy were ghosts.'

Other subjects' reproductions involve similar tendencies to elaborate, fill in missing details, provide connections that they cannot remember and so on. One subject in discussing his reproductions with Bartlett explained he principally tried to reproduce the story from 'images, in a visual form of a wide river, of trees on each side ot it, and of men on the banks and on canoes ... At first I thought there must be something supernatural about the story. Then I thought that Ghosts must be a class or clan name. That made the whole thing more comprehensible.' And indeed in this person's reproduction after a fortnight there appears the passage 'He did not know he was wounded, and returned to Etishu (?). The people collected round him and bathed his wounds, and he said he had fought with the Ghosts.' (N.B. the capital G indicating a proper name.) Here the whole element of the supernatural is transformed into something more comprehensible to this particular subject, who also mentioned to Bartlett that the reason the young man went off to the fight was that 'He was pleased and proud because the Ghosts belonged to a higher class than he did himself.'

Bartlett gives a number of other examples of the efforts of his subjects, each showing various common features, but at the same time each very idiosyncratic. As a last example, here is a reproduction after an interval of two and a half years during which the subject claimed not to have thought about the story since his reproductions in the few months following his original reading.

'Some warriors went to wage war against the ghosts. They fought all day and one of their number was wounded. They returned home in the evening, bearing their sick comrade. As the day drew to a close, he became rapidly worse and the villagers came round him. At sunset he sighed; something black came out of his mouth. He was dead.'

Here, as might be expected following the long delay, is a great deal of omission. But also a conventionalization of the phraseology, and some significant alterations, notably that now the warrior dies at sunset — much more appropriate to die when the sun goes down than when it is rising for a new day.

Bartlett's view of these and his numerous other experiments on remembering and perceiving was that information and reactions were organized within schemata. Thus, instead of supposing that a specific event leaves some specific trace, and that whether that event is remembered depends on whether or not the trace can be reactivated, Bartlett's experiments indicate that 'the past operates as an organised mass, rather than as a group of elements each of which retains its specific character'. Here again we have the notion expounded in the previous chapter that properties of mind emerge from the organization and interaction of parts, not as collections of the parts themselves.

'Schema', Bartlett explains, 'refers to an active organisation of past reactions, or of past experiences ... all the experiences connected by a common interest: sport, literature, history, art, science, philosophy and so on ... There is not the slightest reason to suppose that each set of incoming impulses, each new group of experiences persists as an isolated member of some passive patchwork'.

Bartlett draws from his theory of verbal and perceptual schemata on Head's (1920) *Studies in Neurology*, itself heavily influenced by Hughlings Jackson. Head deals largely with postural schemata in which the results of muscle movements and proprioceptive signals are transformed into an appreciation of postural change 'just as on a taxi meter the distance is presented to us already transformed into shillings and pence ... By means of perpetual alterations in position we are always building up a postural model of ourselves which constantly changes. Every new posture or movement is recorded on this plastic schema ... Such schemata modify the impressions produced by incoming sensory impulses in such a way that the final sensations of position or locality rise into consciousness charged with a relation to something that has gone before.'

For Bartlett too, the schema is the means of organizing experience: 'Remembering is not the re-excitation of innumerable fixed, lifeless traces. It is an imaginative reconstruction, or construction, built out of the relation of our attitude towards a whole active mass of organised past reactions or experience, and to a little outstanding detail which commonly appears in image or language forms. It is thus hardly ever exact, even in the most rudimentary cases of rote recapitulation, and it is not at all important that it should be so.'

In remembering then Bartlett contends that we draw upon first an attitude towards the experience, e.g. in the story of the 'War of the Ghosts', that it was exciting, eerie, or whatever. By 'attitude', Bartlett seems to mean both a matter of feeling or affect, and also it seems, though he is not explicit in this, a general framework for what is being recalled, e.g. that it had to do with warriors and a battle by a river. Minsky (1977) recently has referred to this general setting of structures with which we are familiar as a 'frame'. Secondly, there is the recall of a relatively few highlights, or striking specific details. In the story, for instance, most of the subjects recalled something black coming from the dying warrior's mouth. It is, Bartlett contends, from the attitude and general setting, plus the few significant details, plus the subject's own individual and social 'general knowledge' of the way the world is put together that the experience is reconstructed. Somehow from the few details and the general setting the person infers what must have been the case. Indeed, Bartlett reports that subjects simply given certain outline materials but who have not read a specific story produce constructions which are remarkably similar to his remembering subjects' reconstructions.

What seems to happen is that the general attitude remains

and the construction is a justification or rationalization of how it must have been produced. This, of course, is a rather provocative view of human cognitive processes. Schemata bear an uncanny resemblance to prejudices. The proposition is that through schemata we not only remember our experiences, but perceive and make sense of experiences in the first place. Among the several reasons why Bartlett's work is sometimes spoken of slightingly by experimental psychologists is that this may seem to offer a rather demeaning view of human mental processes to people who would prefer them to be characterized by accuracy and strict logic. Another view (rationalization) of why psychology has been largely dominated by the study of rather isolated responses to meaningless materials in impoverished environments, is that the idea of the schema is much too vague to be able to characterize, let alone to serve as the basis for hard scientific discoveries.

Recently, however, interest in Bartlett's type of approach has been renewed, both by experimentalists, and by people trying to construct computational schemata, or representations. Here, for instance, is a neo-Bartlettian experiment by Bransford and Franks (1971). They created four 'ideas' each of which could be decomposed into four constituent sentences. Examples of complex 'idea' sentences were 'The scared cat running from the barking dog jumped on the table'; and 'The old car pulling the trailer climbed the steep hill'. This last idea, for instance, could be restated in four simple sentences: 'The car was old; 'The car pulled a trailer'; 'The car climbed a hill'; 'The hill was steep'. Sentences containing two of these constituent parts could be created, e.g. 'The old car climbed a hill'. Similarly, sentences containing three constituents could be generated. What Bransford and Franks did was to read to their subjects twenty-four sentences, six generated from each of four basic 'ideas'. From each of the basic 'ideas' were two sentences with one constituent, two with two constituents and two with three constituents. On presentation of each sentence the subjects had to answer a simple question, like 'Did what?'

About four or five minutes after all twenty-four sentences had been delivered subjects were then read another twenty-four sentences, two with one constituent, two with two, one with three and one with four from each of the basic 'ideas'. None of the sentences were the ones they had heard at the first reading, and in addition some were mixtures of the 'ideas', e.g.

'The dog jumped on the old car', or even variations of the basic 'ideas', e.g. 'The scared cat ran from the barking dog which jumped on the table'. These were called 'noncase' sentences. Subjects simply had to say whether they had heard each sentence in the original reading (old) or whether it was new, and rate their confidence in each decision. The results were that for the sentences drawn from the original four 'ideas' subjects uniformly thought they had heard the sentences containing all four of the constituents before. They were progressively less sure that they had heard sentences with three and two components, and very unsure as to whether they had heard the sentences with one component or not. Also they were sure that they had not heard 'noncase' sentences with any number of components. Thus, despite the fact that these subjects had never actually heard any of the complete 'ideas' with four constituents, these were the sentences that they were almost completely sure that they had heard before. In another experiment in the series, where both old and new material was presented for the subject to judge, a similar result occurred, again with sentences being rated as 'old' with progressively more certainty the higher the number of constituents, but with no difference between the sentences that the subjects had actually heard and the ones they had not.

Here, although somewhat confined in the corset of present-day experimental technique, is a recognizably Bartlettian experiment. The subjects first have to make sense of their input, that is, translate it into some meaningful schematic form. Then when it comes to remembering, this schema is used to generate what the input must have been like. What is important, i.e. the meaning of the events described, dominates the recall. The specific forms of words do not.

Clearly 'memory' is involved in nearly all our activities, particularly the more complex ones. Maybe this is what prompted psychologists to study memory as such. But studying it by having subjects learn lists of words tells us very little about the important processes involved. If, as Bartlett and Bransford and Franks argued, remembering is dominated by 'the effort after meaning', then we can study it best in contexts where there is meaning. One should not suppose that meaningfulness can be removed from experimental material so that subjects will exhibit pure memory in tightly controlled experimental conditions which eliminate the variability of the ways in which people make sense of the world. Rather, people seek for meanings even in the meaningless.

It is probably safe to say that in every psychological experiment, even the simplest in which a subject is told to press a button when a light comes on, the subject is trying to make meaningful sense of the situation. One of the kinds of sense he or she makes of it is to conceive it as some more or less elaborate scientific test or exam: 'How well did I do?' It seems possible that the more the experimenter strips down the situation to remove meaningfulness and impoverish the experimental setting, the more uncontrolled (from the experimenter's point of view) will be the meaning that the subject projects into the situation. Thus, rather than creating context-free situations for investigating pure memory or whatever, the experimenter might be creating exactly the opposite, i.e. situations which he or she thinks are carefully controlled, but in which one can have no idea what the subjects make of them. If the kind of meaning a subject ascribes to a situation affects what he or she does, then clearly the impoverishment of the experimental setting until it acts as a sort of Rorschach blot for meanings can have exactly the opposite effect from that desired.

This is not to say that the notion of careful experimental technique in which one varies one condition at a time to investigate its effect is valueless in psychology. But if people make sense of things according to their context, and according to what they individually bring to the situation, then the idea that a particular mental process can be studied 'in isolation' is at least questionable.

Moreover, we seem to have again in the 'stripped down' experiment, the idea that mental processes are a collection of parts whose individual properties sum to make a complex whole. It could alternatively be, as I am arguing in this book, that it is from interaction and context that the properties of mind arise. This is partly why it often proves very difficult, or impossible, to determine the one particular way in which people accomplish some psychological task. Ways vary, both in one person in different contexts and between people.

Perhaps the single general conclusion that can be drawn from the very large amount of work in 'Cognitive Psychology' since the publication in 1967 of Neisser's paradigmatic book with that title is that if one confronts a person with a task in an experiment, he or she will find a plausible way of fulfilling the experimenter's demands. But the way in which he or she does that task may bear little similarity to performance in apparently similar tasks, in which the question asked of the subject was only slightly different. In other words, people have a very flexible set of strategies and will find one, or construct one, for doing the task required of them. This, of course, is upsetting because what experimenters would have liked to find is not a range of strategies, but *the* way in which subjects recognize letters, or remember text, or whatever regardless of context. But this is exactly the kind of answer which has been so elusive.

As an illustration of this curious experimental impasse, consider the question of assigning a stimulus event to a category. We can be thought to make classification judgments when we recognize a friend, read a word out loud, judge the colour of a traffic light and so on. So compelling has been the idea of behaviour-driven classificatory responses that (as discussed in chapter 4) a wide theoretical structure for behaviour has been founded upon it. Irrespective of the usefulness of particular theoretical formations, classification certainly seems to be an important process in the scheme of mental events.

An early proposition of interest with regard to the performance of classificatory tasks is Hick's Law (1952). Hick found that with a number of equally discriminable stimulus lights, and an equal number of response keys, each to be pressed with the finger that was resting upon it, choice reaction time increased linearly as the set of stimuli increased from 1, to 2, to 4, to 8. In other words, reaction time was a linear function of the number of binary choices required to categorize the stimulus. This seemed to be an interesting result, suggesting a certain type of organization of processing. If reaction time is an index of the number of operations required to do a particular task, it seemed to rule out the idea that each each stimulus was checked successively against each possible category, which would have resulted in reaction time being linearly proportional to the number of stimuli. And it also seemed to rule out the possibility of making the categorization by a number of parallel channels between stimulus and response. This would have predicted reaction times independent of the number of stimuli.

However, Leonard (1959), by presenting the stimuli as

vibrations of the response keys rather than lights, did find reaction times to be roughly the same, independently of the number of alternatives, and so did Mowbray and Rhoades (1959) using Hick's original type of display, but giving their subjects a great deal of practice. In these 1959 experiments, one might, therefore, wish to regard subjects' performance as involving the ability to process stimuli in parallel.

Using a not very different categorization technique, that of having subjects remember a small set of items (usually letters or digits), and requiring them to press a button with one hand if a flashed stimulus was in that target category, and with the other hand if it was not, Sternberg (1969, 1975) found a quite different result. Reaction time was an almost exactly linear function of the number of items in the target set. From this it was supposed that subjects made a serial and exhaustive search through the set of items held in their memory, trying to match each in turn with the stimulus. Needless to say, in the rash of experimental data published following Sternberg's results, slight changes in procedure have produced deviations from the linear function, and the rather clear theoretical implications of the data became muddled. Thus, having the members of the target set distinguished by physical features from those of the set of non target items allows the search through remembered items to be performed in parallel (Marcel, 1970), and so does having the target set belonging to one category, e.g. digits, and the non-target items belonging to another, e.g. letters (Simpson, 1972). Moreover, in another choice reaction time task, that of visual search through printed lists of letters, Neisser (1964) found that searching for any of three targets takes no longer than searching for one and the apparent rate of scanning of items is an order of magnitude faster than that found in Sternberg's task.

One can draw a number of conclusions from such experiments (and there is a huge literature on these reaction time and classification tasks). Apart from supposing that each subject is trying to make his or her own meaningful sense of the task, one can also conclude that in any such experiment one is investigating the characteristics of performance of subjects in that particular task, with some given degree of practice, and a particular set of instructions. Generalizations can be made about such matters as the effect of practice, but these do not always help us to understand the mechanisms underlying the classificatory performance, because rather trivial variations of the task seem to allow quite separate strategies to be brought into play by the subjects. One might in that case conclude that human classifications were based on a bundle of special performance mechanisms put together with no very general unifying principles. This conclusion, if correct, would tend to vitiate a good deal of experimental effort, because the purpose of taking psychology into the laboratory is not actually to study reaction time, or retention of lists of nonsense syllables or the mistakes made in recognition of briefly presented items, but to use these techniques to comprehend some principles of memory or perception or whatever in some fashion that will generalize to outside the laboratory. If all we are doing in setting up a scientific laboratory task is to find out how people perform in that particular task, then there is little reason why people other than other experimenters studying exactly the same task should take any interest in any results which emerge. Indeed, if we encase the subject in such tight experimental confines as to constrain his actions entirely into some particular mode, then we run the risk not only of studying behaviour that is so unlike the normal as to tell us little of any general interest, but we also specify the nature of the results before the experiment is even done. And yet even this is unsuccessful because people are inventive, and there is usually more than one way of doing a particular task.

This certainly does not mean that the laboratory should be abandoned. Without scientific observation and experimental method, we might continually assign causal significance to inappropriate events (e.g. Schweder, 1977). One of the principles that seems to emerge, however, is an extraordinary flexibility of human behaviour. This is not necessarily what the psychologist usually means by learning. It includes the fact that in perception the visual scene can apparently summon up from the brain very different interpretations or meanings depending on both personal and external contexts. We can look through a window and see that there are people outside, or perhaps recognize them as friends, or see from their dress and movements that it is a cold day, or from the way they are walking that it is the time of coming home from work. It is this flexibility which is also exhibited in the series of experiments on categorization. Although experimenters conducting a series of experiments may have had in mind a single process, e.g. of classification or recognition, and may have thought that reaction time, or some other measure of the limitation of performance, might tell them something about its characteristics, what emerges rather is a lack of any fixed measurable limitations in this behaviour. As in perception, slight changes in the context of the categorization task produce different results.

Because of the slightly different demands of each task, subjects will perform each in a somewhat different fashion, and it may, therefore, be difficult to find in general *the* limits of behaviour or *the* mechanisms of classification. Indeed, in general, people do not tolerate limitations of their behaviour, but invent both internal (mental) and external ways of overcoming them. Neither do they typically like to perform near the limits of their abilities.

In classical times an 'artificial' aid to memorization of speeches was invented. This involved placing mental images in a series of places in an image of a well-known building. The method grew up as part of the art of rhetoric (Yates, 1966). Nowadays we prefer external aids such as written notes when making speeches. The inventiveness of people and particularly in making instruments that extend human abilities should be a continual reminder that in seeking to understand the brain we are not going to be able to use only those same techniques as might be appropriate to finding out how fixed and uninventive machines like clocks or radio sets work. Not only do we invent tools to supplement our own abilities but we can invent new and better ways of doing things without tools. Moreover, the existence of our own artefacts supports yet newer and successively more powerful ways of thinking. Just as the Greeks used buildings, the most impressive artefacts available as aids to organizing their thoughts, so in later times did other artefacts assist human thought and understanding, right up to today when the computer now acts both as a major extension of our own thought processes, and also as a metaphor or model for understanding our own brains.

Because of the flexibility and creativity of mental processes we will presumably never be in the position of being able to predict exactly a person's behaviour at a particular time. That kind of prediction may be appropriate to physical science and is evidently demonstrated in the sending of rockets to the moon. But for brain research different kinds of testing for hypotheses are necessary. We need to find not only what particular neural processes result in some given behaviour, but what principles make whole classes of behaviour possible.

Summarizing the last few pages, it seems that people when confronted with material which they have to perceive or remember do a number of things. They try to make sense of it, and that sense will include the whole context in which the material is presented, whether or not the experimenter takes steps to eradicate context. The making sense, or the effort after meaning, is affected by culture, and can be highly individualistic. Simply impoverishing the experimental situation gives no guarantee of reducing this individual variation. On the other hand, most subjects are both eager to do well and to please the experimenter, so they typically try to find some way of doing the tasks set as well as they can. This can involve creating strategies which will make the task easier for them. In the situations of great uncertainty that experimenters often create when they are trying to probe the limits of performance, this can take the form of trying to pick up all kinds of little clues (cheat) to get to grips with a task which it is impossible to do perfectly.

In other words, human performance is characterized by a creative, flexible effort after making meaningful sense out of the world. The likelihood is that people thus translate material into their own representations or schemata of the world. These representations will be more or less good for coping with the tasks in hand, and typically people will go on creatively modifying their representations, and perhaps improving their performance.

If this is true, then what is needed in psychology are theories of how representations are constructed and modified. It is here that the attempt to create artificial intelligence becomes important. In so far as we depend for ways of thinking on our own artefacts, we may now wish to entertain more sophisticated theoretical proposals about the brain. We might, for instance, regard memory as a problem of storage, and start thinking of metaphors or models drawn from the natural world, from artefacts like filing cabinets or libraries, or indeed simple boxes. If storage seems to be the problem, we perform experiments to test how good the storage process is. We look for decay (like a melting snowman), or interference (sand on which the footprints of people may cover up the footprints of seabirds). Or we worry about the capacity of a storage box: how many items will it hold? Experiments are then performed to decide among the various possibilities. But the experimental material is often rather trifling; learning and regurgitating lists could be done perfectly by the most rudimentary computer program, or for that matter, by a person armed with a pencil and paper. What many experiments seem to be aimed at finding are the limitations of performance, in tasks that unaided people find fairly difficult, even though they are ridiculously trivial. Since the experiments are set up to examine problems like capacity, or interference effects, these furthermore are all that is found.

However, modes in which we more usually use memory are, for instance, conversation (since an extensive remembered knowledge of the world and the person we are talking to, and the previous conversation, is required to understand sentences, as well as to utter them); or perception (since our knowledge and expectations of how the world is composed are necessary for the interpretation of retinal images). These matters of language and perception are both accomplished easily by people but are in no sense simple; there are as yet (for instance) no computer programs that can perform them anything like as well as people. But one can say that in constructing such programs one will certainly be investigating what memory needs to resemble. And the focus will be not on storage, which is trivial, but on the kinds of meaningful organization and use of remembered knowledge that make language and perception possible.

The use of the term 'metaphor' in this context may seem odd. But I have used it occasionally, both because there seems a strong underlying resemblance between the cognitive processes implied by the words 'metaphor', 'analogy', 'model', 'theory', 'representation', 'schema', and so on, and because in metaphors we can see some of the value of making one thing in our experience stand for something else, which is strictly not that thing. In this literary mode, consider the following poem by Stevie Smith (1957):

> Nobody heard him, the dead man,
> But still he lay moaning:
> I was much further out than you thought
> And not waving but drowning.

Poor chap, he always loved larking
And now he's dead
It must have been too cold for him his heart gave way,
They said.

Oh, no no no, it was too cold always
(Still the dead one lay moaning)
I was much too far out all my life
And not waving but drowning.

Let me, without undertaking a detailed analysis of the poem, point out two levels on which this can be thought of in terms of metaphorical representation. First, there are the marks of print on the page, present in the environment, and we connect these to our own mental representations, not present in the environment, but in our minds, in order to give meaning to the words on paper. Then, at another level, the one for which the term metaphor is more usually reserved, there are the interconnections of different elements mentioned in the poem with some of our, possibly existing or remembered, mental states. So we connect our mental sense of insecurity, perhaps already present as we read, or summoned up by what we read, to the idea of drowning. We connect our fear of being ignored or not understood with waving. The structure in other words, is just the one I have been trying to describe, of events, data, observations in the environment, with which we enter into a relationship by projecting on to them OUR meanings.

In perception, a particular constellation of cues in a retinal image might evoke the schema of a causal interaction such as one object knocking another out of the way. So the retinal pattern allows that construction to be projected on to the environment to make sense of it. Why? Because only in our own mental processes are the rules, and knowledge, and inferences contained, to make meaningful sense of the external event. In the symbolic representations, which emerge as properties of certain structures, are contained procedures concerned with what we might do about it, or what we might want to do about it.

And, just as in the poem, there are other levels beyond that of understanding the words and sentences, so too we find that there is not just perception or remembering, but our attempts to understand our own perception or memory. Here too we project on to the data which is scattered and incomplete, our conceptions of what it might mean — we try to find theories to make sense of it.

Just as in the poem we use the familiar in an interactive process: a familiar sense of insecurity, to give meaning to the words 'not waving but drowning', so in science we project on to data that which is either familiar and part of our experience (e.g. boxes or filing cabinets) on to observations which are the results of experiments. If the metaphor is not part of our own experience (e.g. if we have no personal sense of insecurity), it won't work. If the scientific metaphor, e.g. an equation, is not familiar it won't work for us. And so there is a choice of using that which is already familiar, but which may be feeble like the box as a metaphor for memory. Alternatively, it may need some new experience on our part to acquire it, like mathematics for physics, or computer programming for psychology, or if we are to see perception as a process like doing science, some experience of doing science. And, moreover, the data, when interpreted, can give further content to our experience: the experiment informs the theory, the words 'not waving but drowning' help to give form to our sense of insecurity, or of being misunderstood.

Returning to memory, aided by metaphors like the box, our theoretical explanations of remembering will be directed precisely to performance of boxes, namely containment and storage. With more sophisticated analogies such as filing cabinets we think about indexing and retrieval. But though the container is familiar and well understood, the brain is substantially more sophisticated than any kind of container. One aspect of the importance of computers is the whole new range of metaphors and analogies we can construct. And that is one reason why using computation as a symbolic medium in attempts to create artificial intelligence seems important to the development of our understanding. Perhaps most understanding requires analogy and metaphor. For an understanding is our own cognitive model of what is in common between the two structures or processes that are compared in an analogy or metaphor. With feeble and stereotyped artefacts with which to compare our brain, then just so feeble and stereotyped will our conceptions of brains be.

One most important step that has already been taken in investigating the notion of representations and schemata is that of the attempt to write computer programs that exhibit some of the properties of perceiving visual scenes, and understanding English sentences. The task turns out to be difficult without creating in the program organizations of knowledge corresponding exactly to schemata.

Mental processes based on schemata or representations of knowledge can be recreated in computers, and properties such as understanding (albeit of a simple kind) do emerge from such interacting elements. Clearly, in the computer the elements are simple transistors and so on. But equally clearly the computer can be rightly said to have, e.g. in Winograd's (1971) program, some knowledge about the world and the ability to use it in understanding the sentences it is offered.

The idea that representational properties of mind can emerge from physical elements, and that properties emerge from the interactions between parts rather than being located in the parts themselves can seem mysterious. Here is a typical complaint, in this case made by Sutherland (1975) in a review of Thorpe's book *Animal Nature and Human Nature* (1975).

> In arguing for an antireductionist, emergent view of mind he fields the standard team of obscurantists: Koestler, Polanyi, McKay, Eccles, Dobzhansky, Weiss, Hardy and Teilard de Chardin. His eleven is made up by enrolling two new players, Chomsky and Popper, and by using a theologian (Hick) as long stop. With the exception of the two beginners, these players proceed to throw around terms like 'emergent', 'consciousness', 'determined', 'free-will', 'wholes-greater-then-the-sum-of-their-parts', and so on ... The players have such an enjoyable time tossing the ball to one another and cheering each other on, that they seem quite to have forgotten to notice the opposition. Nevertheless, they make their opponents' task very difficult, since the game is played with no rules or definitions ...

It is not clear from Sutherland's review who the opposition are, or how helpful the cricket match metaphor is. However, I hope I have made clear in this and the previous chapter that notions of emergence are not necessarily obscurantist. They may be complex. Indeed, interactive effects almost by definition require complex organizations. But if they can be demonstrated in computers, they need not seem so mysterious.

Furthermore, our minds may not be good at grasping such interactive processes and the properties which emerge. This again is why the computer as an extension of our own mental processes is important. One way of coming to appreciate how properties of the attribution of meaning do emerge from interacting components is to write or follow a program which generates or understands English sentences, or which processes a simple picture. In the next chapter I shall try to explain in some detail a program, which works on the basis of cues evoking schemata. as a metaphor for perception.

7 *The unconscious inferences of perception*

Though Lashley thought that the way of understanding mind was to concentrate study on the brain, he was hampered by this approach. He argued against the use of analogies for brain mechanisms but in retrospect it seems that his greatest hindrance was precisely the lack of suitable analogies or metaphors for the processes which he rightly regarded as fundamental.

With computers, which bear comparison with brains in the nature of their component processes, in their dependence on a multiplicity of these basic processes, in their flexibility, in their power of representation and in their uses of knowledge, we can now construct metaphors for mind which far surpass anything we have had hitherto. Using these metaphors it seems that we can perhaps more easily understand the basis of the brain's resistance to damage of its parts, the ability of perceptual systems to operate with fragmentary and degenerate input, the ascription of meaning to events, and the nature of intelligent action within the terms of a coherent theory. It is one of the arguments of this book that it is from the standpoint of well-developed psychological theory that the physiological problems are best tackled.

At this stage I will give a description of a particular computational embodiment of a theory of visual perception and then return to physiological and psychological matters. Consider the following task: seat yourself in front of a table and using only vision produce a description of the objects on the table, their shapes and their relationships in the layout of three-dimensional space, as well as their individual positions and orientations to a sufficient accuracy so that you could, for example, reach out and pick any one of them up or say how the scene would look from the other side of the table. This is, of course, the kind of thing that we do implictly whenever we see. We also do more than that; we perceive the functional significance of some relationships, e.g. the teapot lid on the teapot, the knife and fork ready to have a plate placed between them, and so on. In some moods too we seem to experience the presence of objects themselves in an intense way; perhaps our perception of them has been transformed by a particular painter, or they have some particular signficance for us personally.

One method, therefore, of getting to grips with this problem of perception is to start with, say, a camera, or other imaging device; take a picture of the scene, containing, say, children's toy building blocks on the table, and to write a computer program which accepts the picture and returns a description of the scene. In setting ourselves this task, it turns out that all of the problems of reliability in the face of fragmentary input, of reliability of the whole process despite unreliability of the components, as well as of the nature of memory and intelligence, need to be tackled and moved towards some understanding. But they are not tackled because these are processes that are peculiar to man or certain animals, but because these issues are fundamental to the process of seeing in any moderately complex environment. By setting the task of creating a theory that can accept 'real world' data, and by its own processes generate some behaviour, we can make sure that the theory really is a theory about how real behaviour could be produced.

SPECIFICATION OF THE TASK

The nature of perception is that it is an interpretive task requiring a complex and intelligent inference system to undertake it. It has been thought by many people interested in perception of shape and form that the process was essentially one of classification, perhaps following transformations of various kinds. It has been thought of as a detection of aspects of shapes or patterns that would identify them as members of particular classes, e.g. triangle, square etc. Although people and animals can perform such perceptual classification tasks, these are not representative of the perceptual process as a whole. In fact, to suppose that perception is basically a process of pattern classification, is precisely to say that it is based on the reflex theory of behaviour. Stimuli are identified in order to make the appropriate responses. This seems both demeaning and misleading.

The essence of the process is different. It is that given an input which is a succession of not particularly high fidelity, two-dimensional images on the retina, pictures if you like, for which the only parameters are brightness (and colour coding) of points in the array, we must infer the nature and layout of the world with which we are to interact behaviourally and with particular purposes. That is to say, what we experience is ourselves in a setting, say, a room. We experience the layout of the room, its objects, a chair that we might sit on, a coffee cup from which we might drink etc., and we also experience various attributes and relations of these objects, that the table is dirty, or that the washing up needs to be done. The experience of the world in which we live seems so vivid that some authors (e.g. Gibson, 1966) claim that the perceptual experience is direct and flows immediately from what he calls the higher order variables in the visual display, particular patterns of retinal stimulation. Yet we must notice that this is a world of objects which might have uses that might fit with our purposes, of people with whom we might interact, of space in which we might move. It is a world of possibilities for action, described by us and seen by us, in terms of the ways we might interact with it.

In other words, the way we see is in terms of our human purposes in the environment. Yet what is given on the retina is not that. It is anything but that. It is simply a set of excitations, of a two-dimensional array of receptors. The problem then is to take this set of excitations, infer what objects in what kind of layout these might betoken, create in the mind a representation of these objects in their layout. It is this representation, or model of the world and the results of the inferences which can be made within it, which we experience; not the world itself, and certainly not the patterns of excitation on the retina. In so far as perception does allow classification, e.g. recognizing a teacup, it is not so much that we are classifying a pattern or shape in the retinal image, the teacup stimulus, and that it then triggers the response 'teacup', or the related responses of drinking. We infer the presence of a teacup, of a particular kind in a particular place, and we do actually see the cup. We don't see the array of receptor activations as a pattern of light, or indeed as a stimulus. We see it as a teacup, and experience the teacup, and we do not necessarily 'respond'. The understanding of the significance of the cup and the inferences connected with it, allows a whole universe of possible actions.

This, then, is the problem of perception: the processes that Helmholtz (1866) called unconscious inference that allow us to create in our minds a representation which we experience of what it is like out there, given a fragmentary, changing two-dimensional set of receptor excitations.

One obvious way we have at the moment of evolving or testing a formal theory of perception is by creating an artificial perceptual process. We might otherwise think that all the brain had to do is to look at the picture on the retina, somewhat as we look at a photograph, or if we are not misled by that fallacy, then we probably will be by some other one. To avoid fooling ourselves we need to create an artificial process that will see, to act as the formal theory. We need to externalize the process in order to discover it, in order to give ourselves analogies or models for understanding our own perception. A computational model can meet the criterion of taking a real world input, and working under its own steam to produce outputs corresponding to behaviour. Furthermore, the nature and difficulty of the problem task of accepting two-dimensional images, and inferring a description of a three-dimensional layout of objects, is sufficiently tough that in order to fulfil the specification at all, at least some of the important problems which the brain has had to meet will have to be met, principles for coping with them will have to be discovered. Analogies and metaphors for perceptual processes will necessarily be created, so that we can better think about the nature of our own perception.

One important component in understanding the nature of perception is a proper understanding of the domains through which the interpretation process has to pass. In the analysis of a scene we have to start with a retinal image or equivalent, and amongst other things, infer a three-dimensional layout of objects. To do this we have first to form descriptions of the retinal image, the terms appropriate for describing the relevant entities in the domain of two-dimensional picture-images. In other words, there must be a specification of the relative positions of picture points (a Cartesian co-ordinate system is just one way of doing this), a specification of whether particular points or sets of points in this array have special characteristics (as they do in the retina where there are at least three sets of receptors of differential sensitivity to the wavelength of light) and a specification of the brightness value at each picture point. The only descriptions of the retinal image are in terms of these specifications. Other imaging devices, e.g. photographic or television cameras, are similarly restricted. Descriptions in the picture point domain are only in terms of picture points and their properties and their relations.

We might, however, imagine another domain of lines, brightness boundaries, and regions. By operating on the picture in various ways we might translate the description from one in the domain of picture points to one in terms of lines and regions.

In turn, these lines and regions can be interpreted as indicating the presence of various entities in another domain, say, the domain of object parts. Thus a line might be an edge where two surfaces meet, or a crack, or a thin object like a piece of wire, or a thin mark made by a pen. A picture region might be the surface of an object, an area of shadow, or a highlight, the outline of a whole object, or an area painted in a particular colour. Again, there is a distinct domain in which there are particular entities, with particular attributes or properties, and capable of entering into particular relationships with each other. This domain is closer to the world in which we live, and indeed we do 'see' the entities in this domain, the parts of objects if we want to. But there are still other domains.

The object domain might be thought of as one in which the objects and people we see have attributes of size, colour etc., and are related in space. But then there is a further domain of function involving the relation of objects to the purposes we might have with them. Even for some of us there may be yet another domain of people with whom we can relate in a non-object-like way. It is clear, however, that we can also see people as objects. Putting it another way, the whole of perception is involved, as Wittgenstein (1953) argued, with 'seeing as': seeing something, 'we see it as we interpret it'. Thus translation between domains or interpretation of one entity as signifying another becomes possible. Table 1 (from Sutherland, 1973) gives a schematic description of some of the entities, attributes and relationships in a number of visual domains.

There are at present no computational systems that accept the equivalent of retinal images, and are capable of the full range of expression in the domains indicated in the table. Nevertheless, there are several programs available which operate, albeit in a very restricted universe of toy building blocks, somewhere among the domains of picture points,

TABLE 1

Domains involved in scene analysis

Domains		*Entities*	*Attributes*	*Relationships*
Picture	*Points*	points	brightness	next to, above, left of, collinear
	Lines	bars, picture-edges, end, mid-point, vertex	brightness, length, width, orientation	Join, intersect, collinear, parallel
	Regions	regions, vertex, boundary	shape	inside, adjacent
Scene	*Surfaces*	surface, edge, corner, shadow	shape, tilt, albedo	convex, concave, behind, connected
	Bodies	cube, wedge	3-D shape, albedo	on top of, behind, supported by
Object	*Objects*	chair	wooden, comfortable	providing support for human bottom
		person	cheerful, angry	Looking at, hitting, sawing

picture elements, object parts and objects, and these already indicate a number of important principles.

Before describing a representative program it will be helpful to have in mind some of the more important of these principles.

1 *Descriptions*

The programs operate basically by forming descriptions in the different domains. A description, typically a structural description, is one which expresses the relationship between entities in a given domain, and expresses the attributes and properties of the various entities. To move to a higher domain involves taking a description in the lower domain and interpreting that as indicating the possible presence of entities with particular properties and relationships in the higher domain, which then must be described in the language appropriate to that higher domain. Thus a description in the domain of picture elements, which might involve lines of particular orientations and lengths enclosing particular polygonal regions, needs to be interpreted into a description in the domain of object parts involving surfaces bounded by edges. The difficulty arises because there are no simple mapping processes to take, e.g. lines into edges. Lines are very ambiguous and can only be disambiguated by context, i.e. by using large parts of the description, and by everything else one knows about the particular situation. Fig. 7.1, prompted by Wittgenstein (1953) and taken from Oatley (1972), illustrates the ambiguity of a region bounded by three lines.

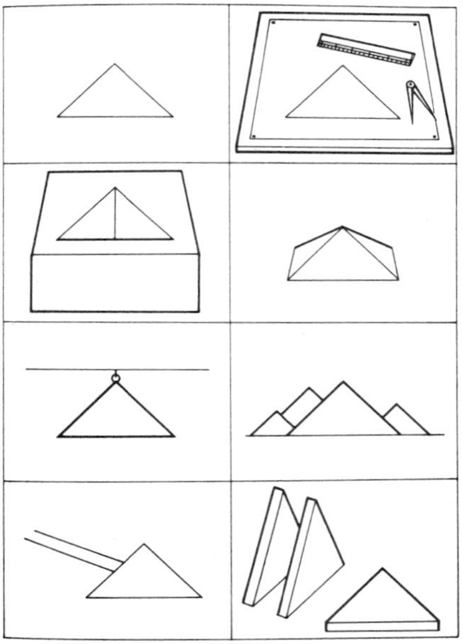

Figure 7.1 Multiple interpretations of a triangle: different contexts enable one to see it as many different things (after an idea of Wittgenstein, 1953; from Oatley 1972).

2 *Heterarchy*

Although it is convenient to think of domains both as separate and ordered from lower to higher, both the separateness and the order to some extent are misleading. In particular, any attempt to move only in one direction from lower to higher domains will be very likely to fail. In the formation of a description at any level both the description from lower domains, and hypotheses from higher domains need to be mobilized. A flexible control structure in which at any point anything relevant that one knows drawn from anywhere else is desirable. Higher level interpretations may be so powerful as to force apparent changes in even the lowest domain, e.g. the cognitive contour phenomenon can be thought of as a perceived brightness gradient forced by an apparent interposition of an object on a background, see fig. 7.2, where 'edges' can be 'seen' despite lack of local evidence.

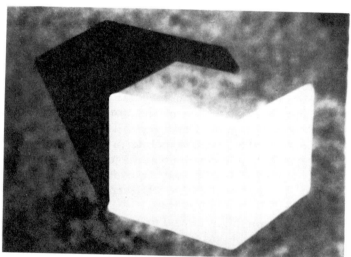

Figure 7.2 Hallucinatory cube: edges can be seen despite lack of local evidence. The photo is actually of 3 cut-out pieces of flat cardboard, (from Clowes, 1973).

3 *Theories and knowledge*

In order to make interpretations at all the program must have some theory of relevant processes within which to make the interpretation. Thus minimally a perceptual program needs to embody explicity or implicity some theory of the image forming process whereby objects in a 3-D layout related to a light source produce a 2-D image projected by a lens system. Furthermore, in order to form hypotheses the program must have, either implicitly or explicitly, some knowledge of what its input could be seen as, i.e. it needs to know in advance what kinds of entities exist in various domains, what properties they have, and what kinds of relations they can enter into.

4 *Cues and hypotheses*

In order to avoid massive inefficiency of the vast searching processes that such complex problem-solving systems can get into, the programs need some ways of being able to invoke high level schemata as easily as possible. Thus one finds that certain arrangements of entities in lower domains can act as cues. And these cues specify or address particular higher level operations, procedures, schemata, or as Gregory (1973) calls them, 'hypotheses', which can then be pulled down to articulate and interpret a description in a particular way.

Armed with these principles (and others have emerged also) we can now study a particular program.

The most important basic program is probably that of Roberts (1965). The program accepts a single 2-D digitized picture of a scene containing polyhedral objects, and entertaining a sort of cubist vision of the world sees it as being composed of prototype objects, the 3-D characteristics of which it knows. It then displays its interpretation of the scene on the visual display of the computer and generates an in-depth rotation of the picture in a way equivalent to an observer walking all the way round the 3-D scene and back to the starting point.

Roberts' program might be said to have three parts, the first accepts a photographic print of a scene, digitizes it and then attempts to deliver a line drawing of it. The second part accepts this line drawing, and by using internal 3-D prototypes or models which it can stretch and rotate tries to segment the 2-D picture into parts that correspond to projections of its 3-D models. Finally, if the program can see the picture as a projection of some arrangement of its 3-D prototypes, it then constructs a 3-D representation of the whole scene from its prototypes, and can, therefore, display what this scene would look like from any angle. I will describe these parts in order in some detail, and following this will make a comparison with known neurophysiological and psychological processes.

ROBERTS' PROGRAM

One scene Roberts treats is shown in fig. 7.3a. From a 4 × 5 inch photographic print, a 256 × 256 picture point version digitized to 8 bits (i.e. 256 brightness levels available for each point) is made (fig. 7.3b: for some reason in Roberts' paper a mirror image transformation has taken place in the digitization

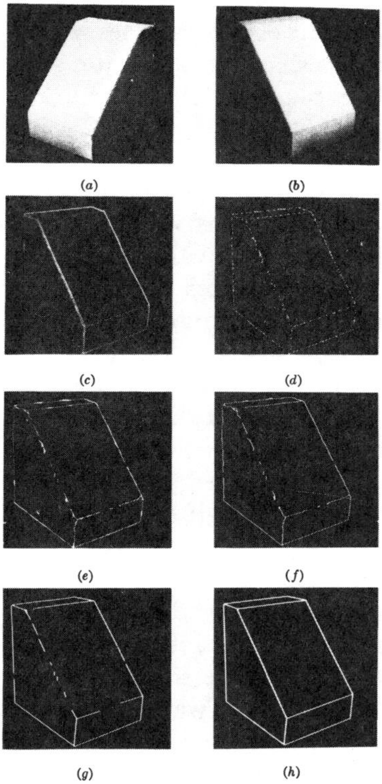

Figure 7.3 Stages in line finding from Roberts' program, (a) is the initial photograph; (h) the final line diagram, and (b) to (g) are intermediate stages, as described in the text (from Roberts, 1965).

process). Then square-roots of the brightness values are taken followed by the application of a differencing operation on these square-root transformed values. This operation is essentially that of finding differences between the square root transformed brightness values of nearest neighbour points in the two diagonal directions, squaring these differences, adding them, taking the square root of this sum and writing in the value of the result into that cell. This is a rather complex type of differencing operation, and Roberts points out that a large variety of alternatives exist. The one he chose was evolved following a series of attempts and, although the computation takes quite a lot of time, Roberts pronounced this well spent in terms of the sharpness of the edges and lines and the reduction of background noise achieved.

Finding differences is the first major step in creating a line diagram for the picture, since the differencing operation selects out a change in brightness values, that is to say, it identifies that set of points in the picture which have large brightness differences, including, one hopes, those brightness boundaries which arise from edges. The relationship between this operation and the equivalent operations that take place in the vertebrate retina will be discussed below.

The next task is to use this differentiated picture to determine the position of continuous lines through the points of large brightness differences. The apparently obvious way of going about this seems to be to select some threshold value such that all the points where large brightness differences occur in the picture stand out above the threshold. One might hope that these would constitute the lines in the line diagram of the scene, while the areas of lower brightness differences are not registered. Roberts remarks that 'the hopelessness of this procedure is easily seen when one looks at a typical picture'. Consider the differentiated brightness values to be represented as height in a sort of three-dimensional contour map of a region of countryside.

> Even a very clean input picture when viewed in this way looks like a bumpy, hilly landscape, with a broken-down stone wall representing the lines, and where some hills are higher than the top of other stone walls. If we imagine the [threshold] level as a flood over this landscape, there is no water level which covers all the hills and yet does not submerge some stone walls. In fact even by adjusting the water level to be optimal for a particular area, a line will look like stepping stones in a rock-strewn brook rather than a smooth dam.

In this striking and apposite image Roberts identifies one of the major problems of perception. The fact that what is offered to the visual system for analysis is a fragmentary, incomplete and messy image even with 'a very clean input picture'. Add to that the poor quality of the optics of the vertebrate eye, the poor quality of the lighting in most scenes which we perceive easily (it is not for nothing that television, films and still photography require carefully arranged lighting). Add also the fact that shadows of retinal blood vessels overlaying the image contribute to the chaos, and one begins to glimpse what a challenging problem perception is. Much of this problem can be overlooked by only studying biological preparations. The problem is not so much to understand how the frog or the cat or man in particular achieve an adequate processing of the image, but how it can be done at all. And setting ourselves the task of doing it computationally is one way of discovering that.

The point is that we are misled by the vividness of our own perceptions into thinking that the outlines of objects, edges, surfaces and so on, are easily seen. Thus we regard line finding as a trivial task, and feel that its essence has been exposed by displaying to animals high contrast spots, edges and lines and finding neurones that respond to these. But if we look at the real world even through our own highly sophisticated process that does segment figure from ground, and identifies the outlines of objects, we can still see how wrong is the simple-minded view that objects have outlines that are present in the image. If we look at almost any ordinary object, the maximum brightness changes such as would be selected by a threshold operation do not necessarily occur at the outlines or edges of the object. If the object is at all shiny, then they will tend to occur in the highlights of reflections. If at all in shadow, then the transition between object and background can involve a much smaller change than a transition from in-shadow to out-of-shadow on a fairly uniform surface of the object. If the object is coloured or has printing or other designs on it then the difficulties multiply. Part of the solution to this is that we have to have well formulated expectations of what kinds of entities we will encounter in three-dimensional domains. The problem is a pervasive and difficult one, not just confined to finding, for instance, straight lines in pictures of plane-sided polyhedra.

Roberts' scheme for finding lines capitalizes on the expectation of being able to find straight lines. Straight lines are precisely those entities in the picture domain which will be significant for seeing a universe composed of plane-sided polyhedra. The question of the relation of this to Hubel and Wiesel's (1959) line segment detectors is clearly apposite and will be discussed below. Roberts' scheme for doing better than the 'flood over the hilly landscape' manoeuvre was to look for local straight-line features of the differentiated picture first, and build up to the determination of long straight lines in a series of steps. This procedure saves time over a process applied uniformly to the whole array, and also can take account of the local noise level over restricted areas, and thus adjust the process to local rather than global conditions.

The initial line segment fitting process starts by finding a brightness difference, and inspecting a 4 × 4 point array around it. Then using a low threshold for each such area try and fit lines with angles corresponding to 0°, 45°, 90°, and 135° from vertical around this point within the 4 × 4 array. If the ratio of the best to the worst fit of these four slopes exceeds another threshold, a line segment is taken to be present, and its exact best direction is calculated. The point, and this best direction are recorded. This process first identifies a region with probable line segment and then determines its orientation.

Line segments are then connected if they are in touching 4 × 4 squares, so long as their directions are within ± 23° of each other. Points left unconnected by this process are eliminated, and the result is a preliminary line drawing of many short lines. The problems with treating this are first that sections of lines are missing, and secondly that some sections may have multiple connections, e.g. where there is a junction of lines, and also where the line is rather wide. To eliminate these blotchy areas and create well-defined junctions, small closed polygons of lines (e.g. triangles and quadrilaterals) are identified. For a triangle the longest line is deleted; a quadrilateral is compressed along its longest axis. Then any spurs connected at only one end are deleted.

By now a picture with relatively clean thin lines has been achieved. But this is not yet an outline drawing of the scene. The program next fits by a least-squares procedure long straight lines to points identified as belonging to short line segments. Starting at any such point the procedure extends the line in one of the two directions defined by the segment until either it meets a point with more than two line segments attached to it, or until some threshold of the mean square error for the fitted line is exceeded. If it finds that the error is exceeded, it backs up until the angle between the computed line and the little line segments is decreased by a factor of 2, and this point usually identifies a junction. The line is then extended in the same manner in the opposite direction and the result is a picture with long fairly accurate lines which have breaks in them, or which meet at junctions. Lines which are still unconnected are now grown at both ends, checking the correlation with the differentiated picture as this is done, and if this growth process results in meeting another line, then the two are joined, otherwise the line segment is deleted. In the final step of what might be called the preprocessing stage another bout of least-squares fitting with the by now longer line segments is undertaken to eliminate any spurious junctions which might have been created by previous manoeuvres. At last for some simple, clean, pictures of matt painted opaque polyhedra without shadows or highlights a line drawing is produced.

The sequence of operations from digitization of the original photograph and to the cleaned up line drawing is illustrated in fig. 7.3(a) to (h). Only at the last stage depicted by (h) has the computer achieved an interpretation of well-defined straight lines which correspond to the edges of the object that we would see. That is to say that despite our own visual impressions of the sequence of pictures in fig. 7.3 the outline drawing of the object is only chieved at the last stage. The fact that we can see any of the pictures (a) to (h) as a quite good representation of an object merely indicates how powerful our own interpretive processes are. But in the digitized picture there are no lines or edges, only picture points of varying brightness. In the differentiated picture, there are no lines, only points where a large difference in brightness occurs. To see these as straight lines the program needs to have an expectation of straight lines. It then proceeds to supply or project this expectation from within, first in the form of small line segments, and later in a linear least-squares fitting procedure. The data in the picture, in a sense, merely guide the program as to where these hypothesized lines should be placed. The data do not actually provide or contain the lines — they are not there in the picture only in the interpretation. Clowes (1973) uses an apt phrase for this kind of process — 'hallucination'. But it is a hallucination which is controlled, or cued by the picture (image) evidence. And it is a process which is effective even in areas of a picture where there are no local brightness gradients at all (see, for instance, the cognitive contour fig. 7.2). This kind of picture begins to give us some slight inkling of the power of the problem-solving processes in vision, and of the conclusion that if we see part of a picture as an entity, then in order to make that interpretation the entity (i.e. the candidate interpretation, the hypothesis or the hallucination) needs to be supplied not from the picture itself, but from the perceiver.

The next part of Roberts' program contains further perhaps even more direct examples of this. As far as table 1 goes the program has achieved a description of the picture in the domain of picture points and interpreted this description into another domain, that of picture elements, i.e. lines. The computer at this stage would in other words hold simply a list of two-dimensional co-ordinate values of the end points of the twelve straight lines in fig. 7.3(h), and this is the description which is offered to the next stage which will try to interpret this collection of lines as solid objects.

Again in order to make the interpretation, the program has to be provided with a set of candidate hypotheses; expectation of what it might encounter. These take the form of the co-ordinate values in 3-D space (since the interpretation of the picture is to be of 3-D objects) of three prototypes or models.

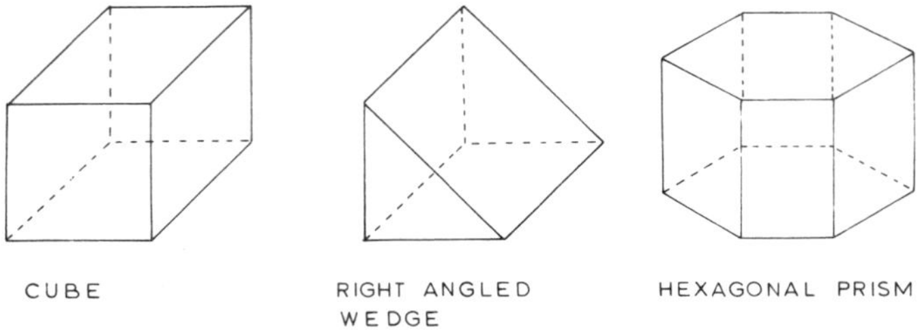

Figure 7.4 Three-dimensional prototypes used in Roberts' program.

The models, illustrated in fig. 7.4, are a cube, a right-angle wedge, and a hexagonal prism. The program has the means of manipulating these prototypes, i.e. stretching or compressing them in any dimension, rotating and translating them. It also has the theory that what exists in its world can be understood to be made up of these prototypes in various elongations or rotations and with complex objects being composed of several of its prototypical models stuck together in some way. It also has a theory of image projection of 3-D objects onto a 2-D surface such as a retina or a photographic plate. Armed with these manipulable prototypes and its theory of projection its task is to see the line drawing as the outline projection of some particular arrangement of its 3-D prototypes. In fact, by using these prototypes it is able to deliver a 3-D description of the objects depicted in the picture.

As well as being of a cubist disposition, the program can be thought of as adopting a kind of Platonic view of the world. Its prototypes correspond to the Platonic ideas, which are reflected in rather corrupted form in the 2-D projection which it accepts. And these ideas happen to be of a cubist kind. Just as Picasso and Braque around 1910 analysed their world into elementary polyhedral solids, so too does Roberts' program.

There are in the next part of the program transformations of the 3-D prototypes, i.e. expansions, contractions, translations and rotations of the prototypes, which are undertaken using a system of matrix algebra with homogeneous co-ordinates. Though this will not be described here in detail, it is in one sense the heart of the computation of this program. Basically it consists of a theory of projection of 3-D objects onto a 2-D surface in an imaging system such as a camera. In the real world any point on an object will have three Cartesian co-ordinate values, say, x, y, and z. In the projection of this point onto a picture it is possible to calculate its picture co-ordinates, say, x^1 and y^1, and Roberts describes a transformation to achieve this, and calls this transformation P. He also has another transformation called R which takes a prototype, also specified in 3-D co-ordinates, and allows rotation, transformation and size change in x, y or z directions. If now he can identify a set of points on the 3-D model that could correspond to points on the 2-D picture, he can inquire whether there are transformations P and R which would project the model points onto the picture points. If so, then the picture could depict the model under the particular transformations found. In other words, the program would have succeeded in seeing part of a picture as a projection of an example of one of the kinds of things it knew existed in its world, i.e. a prototype or model.

The details of the matrix operations which produce the transformations and similarity tests which gauge the success of a particular controlled hallucination need not concern us here. The matters of major psychological importance seem to be not so much in the matrix algebra in which the transformation and matching processes are achieved as in the ways in which these transformation and matching processes are deployed, in the structure of a hypothesis selection and testing procedure.

The program with the set of line definitions first undertakes some list processing and counting operations to determine what polygonal regions there are in the picture. Thus, for instance, in fig. 7.5(A1), the largest polygonal region (apart from the background) is a pentagon, formed by one side of the larger of the two objects depicted. The partly obscured face of the parallelopiped behind it appears in the picture domain as an irregular 7-sided figure. Part of the problem is to interpret that 7-sided region in the picture domain as part of a 4-edged surface in an object domain.

Having found the polygonal regions in the picture (itself a non-trivial task as it turns out), the program next looks for particular sets of such regions. To depict an unobscured surface of one of the prototypes, a region must be either triangular, quadrilateral or hexagonal, because these are the only shapes or surfaces exhibited by the three prototypes used. Roberts calls these three figures 'approved polygons'. The program now looks for particular sets of approved polygons which could select a particular prototype to try and project onto the picture. It tries to discover the existence of a configuration of approved polygons as follows: are there (1) three approved polygons surrounding a point, or if not, (2) two approved polygons on either side of a line, or if not, (3) one approved polygon with a line attached?

These configurational cues allow Roberts to undertake what he calls topological matching, to identify not only which prototype hypothesis to select but which points on it to match to points on the picture. Thus, suppose a point is found on the picture surrounded by three approved polygons (triangles, quadrilaterals or hexagons) the program searches through the models to find an equivalent configuration. Any group containing the cue 'triangle' will immediately select the hypothesis 'wedge'. Similarly, a hexagon is a cue to selecting the hexagonal prism. Three quadrilaterals around a point select the cube, and so on. The program then cycles around the model and the picture to line up the order of the polygons, applies transformations of e.g. expanding or contracting sides of the model to look to see whether a fit can be made (using a least-squares procedure), in which case that part of the picture can be seen as the projection of that particular transformation of the prototype. If this is so, the program then has from the model the information about corners, edges and surfaces of the object that may not appear in the picture because they are obscured by the opacity of the objects. In other words, it has achieved at least part of a three-dimensional description of the scene.

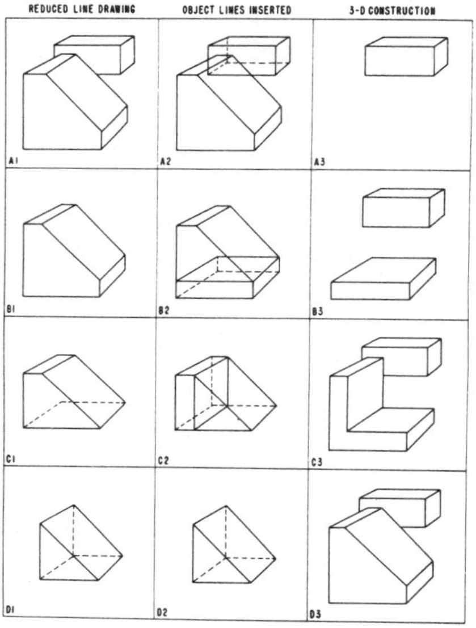

Figure 7.5 Stages in construction of a 3-dimensional scene from a 2-dimensional picture; for description see text (from Roberts, 1965).

The mechanics of this process become clearer in treating a particular example which Roberts gives (see fig. 7.5). Starting with a line diagram corresponding to diagram (h) of fig. 7.3, the program first finds the polygons of the figure. There are seven polygons with interior boundaries; the exterior boundary around the group is found but not used at this stage. The interior polygons consist of one septagon, a pentagon, and five quadrilaterals. No point can be found on the picture which is surrounded by three approved polygons, so the program searches for the somewhat weaker cue configuration of two approved polygons separated by a line. There are, in fact, three instances of this in all cases involving two quadrilaterals. This configuration invokes the cube hypothesis. (This is called first to avoid splitting parallelopipeds up into wedges.) However, when it comes to trying to fit a cube model to the quadrilateral parts of the object nearer to the camera, the program fails to find an unskewed transformation of a cube which will fit. However, for the partially obscured body (further from the camera) it does find a transformation which will fit the two quadrilaterals, by stretching the cube model out sideways.

The program looks to see whether any of the points on this hallucinated projection of the model fall outside the outer boundary of the group of blocks. Line junctions forming T shapes (i.e. with one line stopping at a cross line) are used as evidence for obscuration of one body by another, and these junctions are again used as cues, in this case cues which allow the extension of lines in the projected model to restore (as it were) the obscured edges. This process of adding the edges of the object which are obscured both by the object itself and by other objects is undertaken, as shown in A2 of fig. 7.5. At this stage the program has a firm conception of the nature of the further of the two objects, and all the lines belonging to it are marked as having been used. Notionally, this part can be thought of as being temporarily removed from the picture and put on one side (A3 of fig. 7.5) leaving the remaining part as shown in B1 of the picture.

A new search is now begun on this remaining part. The best that can be found as a cue in this part of the picture (given that neither of the sets of two quadrilaterals separated by a line will produce a model fit) is the weaker one of one approved quadrilateral with an attached line. There are two acceptable instances of this, and the program selects the lower one first, and again goes through the process of projecting its cube model onto this part of the picture. It again adds the unseen lines, and in this case also joint lines of the cube with the rest of this compound object. In other words, it sees this compound object as being composed of a lower part which fits its cube prototype. And this part with its three-dimensional structure is put on one side, see B3 of fig. 7.5.

A similar process is performed for the left-hand side of the object, finding and removing another instance of the projected transformed cube prototype, see fig. 7.5, C1, C2 and C3. Finally, only a wedge is left, which does fit with the wedge model (the back edges having already been determined, this is actually unnecessary) and this is entered into the 3-D description (see D3 of fig. 7.5).

Having now acquired a description of the scene in terms of its 3-D prototypes, Roberts' program has now effectively 'seen' the picture as a set of objects, in 3-D space. Because it holds the 3-D co-ordinates of the corners of the objects it can now re-transform this 3-D description into a 2-D projection from any point of view, and indeed proceeds to show on the computer display what the picture scene looks like from behind, and from other points of view.

Roberts' was the first and in many ways the most interesting of the programs to achieve 'perception' of a visual scene. At this stage it is worth making some fairly detailed comparisons with physiological and psychological understandings of visual perception. I will discuss four main points; the problems of differentiation of the picture images to find regions of maximal brightness change, the problem of the finding and fitting of small straight line segments, the question of the role of cues in perception, and the issue of the manipulation and use of visual schemata.

DIFFERENTIATION AND LATERAL INHIBITION

The work of many neurophysiologists on lateral inhibitory networks is too well known to require any lengthy description here. For more detailed treatments see Ratliff (1965), Cornsweet (1970), Ratliff and Hartline (1974). It is sufficient for the present purposes to describe the common neurophysiological finding of lateral inhibition in the retina, and the main psycho-physical phenomena that are usually associated with it.

Transduction of light energy into an electrical potential takes place with a function which is not linear, but negatively accelerated. That is to say, in an experiment where incident light intensity increases, in a logarithmic scale, say, doubling on each step, the electrical response, rather than doubling increases by a similar amount each time. The transduction function in other words tends to flatten off, indeed as Werblin and Dowling (1969) have shown, it actually saturates at a particular asymptote for a particular receptor. There has been a long argument between the followers of Fechner, who have thought that sensory magnitude, which was supposed to reflect the transduction process, was a precise logarithmic function, and Stevens (1961) who claims that it is a power function. The issue scarcely seems important here. The function in visual receptors is a decelerating one, and this is reflected in Roberts' use of a square root transformation of his digitized brightness data, following Stevens rather than Fechner. What would be more interesting would be to test the actual effect of various transformations on signal to noise problems in subsequent processes. But this was something Roberts did not report.

The next transform that is taken in Roberts' program is again similar to that found in the retina. What has been found (e.g. by Barlow, Fitzhugh and Kuffler, 1953) in vertebrate visual systems by recording from ganglion cells whose axons form the optic nerve is that each cell responds not to absolute light levels, but to differences. A cell has a receptive field (a term used by Sherrington to mean the receptive area within which it could be affected), and within this area the optimal or adequate stimulus is one in which the brightness differs from part to part. In fact, in vertebrates the typical receptive field organization is of a so-called centre-surround kind. A bright area in the centre of the roughly circular field will increase excitation of the cell, whereas a bright annulus occupying the rest of the field will inhibit it. Thus, for maximal effect there must be a brightness difference within the field, for example, with the centre area bright and the surround dark. Half the cells found have the opposite arrangement of being excited by a dark centre surrounded by a bright area. In any case the effect is clearly that of applying a differencing operation. The neurophysiologist's notion of the receptors affecting the ganglion cell in such a way as to produce lateral inhibition, i.e. that receptors on either side of the centre have an inhibitory (or opposite) effect from the centre, is very close to Roberts' transform of taking differences between neighbouring picture point brightnesses and passing on only these differences to the next stage. Ratliff (1965) gives various mathematical models of the neurophysiological process, none of which is exactly that used by Roberts, but the intention and the effect are similar: namely, to produce an output from this stage which is at each point proportional to the spatial change of brightness. The effect is that over regions of uniform illumination no output at all occurs from such a stage, whereas where there is a high contrast brightness contour, a row of cells along that contour is energetically affected.

Lateral inhibition is associated with a number of perceptual phenomena but most importantly with local adaptation. That is to say, over any small region of the visual field there is a mean brightness level, to which the visual system is not responsive. It only responds to changes of brightness value around this mean. This means that the retina can respond to detail simultaneously around very different local mean brightness values in a scene. In contrast, artificial imaging devices have to be set to respond about the mean brightness for a whole view. This means either that photographers often have to arrange the lighting carefully to eliminate deep shadows or bright spots, or if they do not, then the detail in such areas will be obscured.

The problem has a close relationship with Roberts' metaphor of the stone walls in hilly countryside. It is interesting to note that Roberts rejects the apparently most straightforward approach to this problem, i.e. a mechanism of locally adjusting the threshold of the output of the differencing or lateral inhibition stage. In terms of his analogy Roberts argues that 'even by adjusting the water level to be optimal for a particular area, a line will look like stepping stones in a rock strewn brook'. Roberts, therefore, places the onus of his locally sensitive mechanism at the next stage, that of line segment fitting.

It is fair to comment that since Roberts is only dealing with simple photographs of carefully lit scenes, the wide variation of light levels with which the eye can cope is not met. Roberts' refusal simply to have a locally adjustable threshold indicates that there are other possibilities than the lateral inhibition stage for producing the perceptual effect of local adaptation, and that in the eye the lateral inhibition mechanism almost certainly contributes to this valuable property, but does not completely explain it.

Using the metaphor of Roberts' program, the function (and the perceptual phenomena) of lateral inhibition can be seen fundamentally not as finding edges or lines as such, but simply as identifying those points in the picture where large local brightness changes exist. Smaller brightness changes, or variations over large regions, are (neurophysiologically) rejected apparently, perhaps because they will hinder line construction processes, and because they have little behavioural significance. The colour of (say) a painted surface which we see as uniformly bright will not typically exhibit physically equal brightness values; e.g. because of changing distance from the light source, or shadows or highlights. Its seen uniformity is a hypothesis created by higher level inferential processes.

There is an empirical question here which has not yet been answered. It has to do with how far the human visual system relies on entirely global transforms of the visual data starting from the domain of retinal receptor excitations. The power law transformation, and the lateral inhibition transformation can be seen as essentially global processes applied willy-nilly to all retinal images, and to all parts of the image. Ginsberg (1975) makes the case for a great deal of preprocessing of pictures by transforms and spatial filtering operations to extract and enhance significant patterns in pictures. Moreover, Sullivan (Personal communication) has demonstrated a television system which makes a remarkable job of performing local adaptation, by applying a single lateral inhibition transform to the signal coming from the TV camera. Its effect is particularly noticeable where part of the scene is in shadow, such as a televised football match where the grandstand casts a shadow over part of the field. Both players and ball become difficult to see on an ordinary television picture when they pass into that shadow.

The issue is, therefore, not the usefulness of such wholesale transforms, Roberts, Ginsberg and Sullivan all make the case convincingly, but at what point higher level, meaning-based schemata may affect specific interpretations in lower domains. Roberts' program has clear divisions and no interactions between the stages: preprocessing (i.e. power law transform and differentiation), line fitting, model invocation. The latter two are selective: lines, and 3-D stereotypes guided by cues are projected onto parts of the data, the initial transforms, however, are global. We do not know in human vision whether there are such divisions of global and selective processes or if so where the divisions might occur.

LINE FINDING

The reason why lateral inhibition does not completely cope with the local adaptation problem is hinted at by Roberts' reference to 'stepping stones in a rock strewn brook'. The putative line is not continuous, and one stepping stone is very much like another rock. In other words, the line is not actually there in the differentiated picture at all, only in our perceptions of it. The fact that we do not see the equivalent of the rocks in the brook when we look at the world is not that there is a threshold level which will just make the signal of the stepping stones stand out from the noise of rocks, but that some configurations are significant for our perceptions of objects (e.g. colinear points of fairly high spatial change of brightness) and some are not (e.g. randomly scattered points of high spatial change of brightness). Because Roberts knows that straight lines are the significant features of his picture, because straight edges of the polyhedral bodies are depicted by them, he devotes a great deal of the first part of his program to projecting line hypotheses onto the picture. He does not really find lines in the picture, rather his program hallucinates them onto regions of the picture. It is only their positions and orientations which are controlled by the brightness changes of the picture itself. Thus to avoid seeing the rocks in the rock strewn brook, Roberts fits four orientations of line, at 45° intervals over each local area, and only if the ratio of the best to the worst fit here exceeds a certain value does the program 'see' anything in that area at all. If the ratio does exceed a threshold, then this is a good indication of a co-linear set of points, in which case the program supplies a line in that region, and indeed finds the orientation of the line segment which gives the best least-squares fit. Thus it is the program that supplies the lines, not the picture. Even at this 'preprocessing' level perception is a matter of hypothesis and test, not simply transformations of the picture data.

In this context the properties of Hubel and Wiesel's (1959, 1962) so-called simple and complex cells which respond to line segments is obviously relevant. In chapter 1, an argument was put forward that finding that neurones had a particular 'adequate stimulus' did not actually tell us anything about their role in the neuronal mechanism. We would only be able to understand that role within the context of a particular theory that we were entertaining about the process. Thus, if the theory of brains that we were entertaining were basically a reflex one, then the only job of the visual system would be to categorize these patterns as distinct stimuli. The role of Hubel and Wiesel cells, therefore, would simply be as classification elements. If on the other hand we have a theory which supposes that perception is a process of 'unconscious inference' (as Helmholtz proposed), yielding a description of the three-dimensional layout of the world, and descriptions of the people and objects and their spatial inter-relationships in it, and if, furthermore, we can specify some version of such a theory in a formal manner (as Roberts has made a start at), then we will be able to achieve different interpretations of the role of such elements. Just as within the visual system candidate interpretations of the retinal image are supplied from within, so in understanding perception we ourselves have to be able to supply from the overall psychological theory we hold, candidate interpretations to hallucinate onto the experimental data. This seems to be at least one important way in which cognition works.

In any case, Roberts' program provides a different kind of theory within which we can interpret neurophysiological and psychological data. Within this theory we could see Hubel and Wiesel cells as applications of the operations of deciding whether a line segment could be fitted, and if so pass the description of a line segment at a particular place and with a particular orientation. Roberts makes it clear though that this is a very preliminary stage in achieving a description of the figure in terms of lines. Joining up colinear regions with similar orientations is needed, finding corners, deleting small polygonal configurations and spurs, and filling in at least some of the gaps in lines is needed.

Within such a scheme it is interesting to note that the sharpness of orientation tuning of orientation sensitive cells in the cat's cortex (Campbell, Cleland, Cooper and Enroth-Cugell, 1968) is of the same order of magnitude as Roberts' criterion for adjacent line segments being co-linear, namely $\pm 23°$. The properties of hypercomplex cells (Hubel and Wiesel, 1965) may have less to do with forming more complex classifications than with finding end points and junctions of lines. The more recent findings of Blakemore and Tobin (1972) that orientation sensitive neurones are inhibited by differently oriented striped patterns outside their normally defined receptive field area could now receive an interpretation in terms of determining the line continuations.

The difficulty in such analyses is that data collected under some such aegis as interneurones being units of pattern recognition, which classify their input patterns as many neurophysiologists have claimed, will, of course, be of just that kind, i.e. input pattern classifiers. From within this theory classification is all that neurones can be seen to do. Other kinds of event are simply the rocks in the rock strewn brook. This kind of issue argues for the central role of theory in brain research, and for a role of computation and artificial intelligence, not in providing substantive answers, but in increasing the range of theories, models, metaphors or ways of thinking, that we can bring to bear on the problem. At present, as Uttal (1973) points out, rather unsatisfactory relationships between neurophysiological and psycho-physical findings tend to be proposed. I would like to suggest that this in part is due to the dominance of a psychological theory of stimulus classification.

Even so it is significant that Hubel and Wiesel have discovered straight line detectors, not curved line detectors, or blob detectors, or irregular edge detectors. this may be an indication that Roberts' twin strategy of (a) interpreting the picture as composed of lines and (b) supposing that the significant line segments are straight, is not merely appropriate to the restricted world of plane polyhedra. But we will need a good deal more theoretical development beyond Roberts' program to be able to penetrate the problem of less artificial perceptual worlds, either than those projected with high contrast onto screens to neurophysiologically prepared cats, or than those offered for computational analysis.

CUES AS IDENTIFYING SCHEMATA

Leaving the strictly neurophysiological field for the moment, Roberts' program continues to provide us with understanding of why perception is not simply a stimulus classification task. If seeing is in Wittgenstein's (1953) phrase 'seeing as', then the entities that parts or wholes of pictures are seen 'as' depicting must be supplied from within. The data of the picture have the role mainly of controlling where, how far away, and in what spatial orientations and relationships these entities are to be seen.

Two naive strategies exist in parsing (i.e. assigning structure) to input patterns. One is sometimes called 'bottom up', and the other 'top down'. With the 'bottom up' approach, the idea is to start from the elements in the lowest domain (e.g. the picture points of table 1), and gradually work up towards more and more complex interpretations. This contains the difficulty of making a global search through an infinite number of possible interpretations of the patterns, and putting the onus of that guidance on the patterns themselves. The other, 'top down' approach requires that there be well formulated expectations of what the significant things to see in the picture are, before the picture has been analysed. It clearly contains the difficulty of understanding what range of expectations will be adequate to the task of coping with real, as opposed to artificial environments, and of how we can see entirely novel objects at all.

No doubt actual perception involves both 'bottom up' and 'top down' operations, but it is certainly true that if we can identify high level hypotheses early on in the process, an enormous amount of effort is saved. One major problem here is therefore to identify in the picture, or one of the lower domains, configurations which will act as cues to select appropriate high level hypotheses. Thus in Roberts' program the cue to see a line in a particular small region is an above-criterion ratio of best to worst fit among lines fitted at 45° to one another. Yet more significantly the cues to the selection of one of the 3-D schematic prototypes, are particular arrangements of approved polygons in the line drawing: those polygons which could be projections of one of the program's prototypes. In general the higher the level of the hypothesis that can be selected, the better the cue.

In human vision, we are clearly equipped with a rich repertoire of cues for invoking the schemata of people. These operate powerfully to over-ride certain contradictory information in the picture itself, as in Gregory's (1970) demonstration of our being able to see a concave 'face' (e.g. from the inside of a mould) as convex, despite the fact that shadow information is wrong. Schemata also act even to supply information that is not in the pictures at all. Thus Clowes (1973) shows how anatomical and sociological knowledge is needed to interpret parts of a not particularly well printed newspaper picture. Even more strikingly, a particular pattern of relative movements of the arrangement of bright dots shown in fig. 1.3, immediately evokes a perception of a person with lights attached to his or her ankles, knees, hips, wrists, elbows, shoulders and head, walking or performing some other characteristic movement. Johansson (1971) has shown in films that these moving patterns are so powerful in invoking human schemata, that not only can one see a shadowy outline of the of the moving figure (where no brightness information actually exists) but the movements of walking, dancing, doing press-ups etc. are clearly perceived. All that exists on the film are relative movements of lights, which presumably act as cues to the schemata of arms, legs, and other bits of anatomy, and these contain the knowledge that we have about them, and the inferences from that knowledge.

Evidently, the higher the level of the hypothesis a cue can identify the more efficient the process. With schemata for non-human objects too we can see a similar supply of missing information, which is cast in the terms of meaningful objects or events; interpretations in terms of the purposes we have in the world.

Thus from Roberts we can derive a new definition of the psychologist's idea of the cue. It is an arrangement of entities in a lower domain (e.g. the picture) which can be identified within that domain, and which points either to a particular higher level schema such as a cube in Roberts' program, or to some higher level process. For example, the T-junction is a cue for a procedure analysing the partial obscuration of one object by another.

This idea that there are analysable patterns in, for instance, the picture domain which can select high level hypotheses is clearly a very valuable one. Until recently cues were usually taken by psychologists to mean 'depth cues'. However, it is clear that all sorts of cues which invoke higher level hypotheses could exist. Kinetic cues are obviously very powerful. The Johannson (1971) demonstrations are one example. Another is Michotte's (1963) demonstrations of causal perception, in which two dots move with respect to each other, and under some circumstances causation is perceived, e.g. when one dot moves to become adjacent to the second and stops, whereupon the second moves off in the same direction as that of the first. This is seen (under some circumstances) as a causal interaction, with the first spot knocking the second like a shove-halfpenny. Clearly there is something about the spatio-temporal pattern which invokes the hypothesis of a particular kind of causal interaction and we see it 'as' causation: an event important in the interpretations we make in conducting our purposes in the world. Even more complex schemata or hypotheses are invoked by the kind of display used by Heider and Simmel (1944). They made a short cartoon film in which a large and small triangle and a small circle moved around on the screen which also depicted a simple plan view of a hut (see fig. 7.6). People's

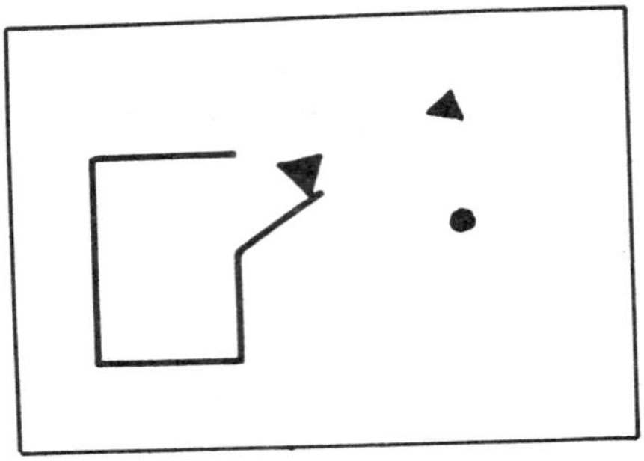

Figure 7.6 Still picture from Heider and Simmel's cartoon movie (from Heider and Simmel, 1944).

descriptions of the movie indicated that they saw various kinds of interactions, ranging from the physical, e.g. hitting, opening or closing a door, to the purely psychological, e.g. chasing, threatening. This display is clearly a very impoverished picture, yet the configurations invoke very complex schemata, many of them of an animate kind. It may be also that the so-called sign-stimuli which evoke particular patterns of instinctive behaviour in lower animals, e.g. Tinbergen's (1951) demonstration that male sticklebacks are induced to perform mating behaviour by being confronted with very crude models of the gravid female could also be thought of as cues rather than stimuli. In this judgment of whether to see this in terms of stimuli or cues, there is, as in other cases of how we see the world, more than one interpretation.

THE NATURE OF SCHEMATA

Bartlett (1932) is the person most closely identified with extolling the virtue of schemata. His work was a reaction against what he saw as the sterility of the tradition in verbal learning stemming from Ebbinghaus, in which everything was sacrificed to the idea of being able to measure aspects of memory. Learning of lists of nonsense syllables was not only artificial to a degree, Bartlett argued, but irrelevant to the real problems of understanding memory. Indeed, if perception and memory are based, as Bartlett supposed on 'an effort after meaning', the learning of nonsense syllables was very much beside the point.

As discussed in chapter 6, Bartlett's theory was that we have mental or cognitive schemata, organizations typically of common-or-garden general knowledge about the world. These organizations of knowledge are dependent on our particular social and cultural background, and also on the particular purposes that we pursue in the world.

Bartlett has been criticized for being too vague, for putting forward a view that was not new and which everyone in some sense understood already, without adding to that understanding, and even for taking a soft option with undefined propositions, rather than grappling with hard formal theories in an attempt to make them less inadequate.

One of the results of writing computer programs to undertake verbal conversation, perception and problem solving has been precisely to give the important concepts which Bartlett saw as necessary a more formal expression. In other words we can now construct and experiment with schemata or structures of knowledge which are addressed by cues, and perhaps understand a great deal more about their properties. Robert's constructive process based on prototypes and a theory of projection is a formal expression of a Bartlettian schema.

Among the important concepts is the idea that schemata, representations or models of the world are more or less good for a particular task. Thus our perceptual schemata of solid objects, spatial layout, support, occlusion and so on no doubt take the form they do because we might want to pick up objects, avoid bumping into them, sit on them etc. Even if it were possible for our naive physical schemata to correspond to that of modern physics, i.e. with space being sparsely occupied by fundamental particles, which are themselves packets of energy, such a schema would be useless for our everyday life. It is not easy to see how interpretations within such a schema would allow us to interact with the world in the ordinary way that we do. In other words particular schemata are appropriate to particular tasks in particular environments.

8 *Degenerate data and reliability of function*

One major problem of psychology, raised by Lashley, and raised again by artificial intelligence is how is it possible to produce complete and integrated percepts and sequences of behaviour on the basis of data from the outside world which is fragmentary and when the components of the brain are unreliable. Lashley's answer was rather unsatisfactory. He continually pointed out what was wrong with other people's formulations, convincingly arguing, for instance, that any version of connecting responses to stimuli was hopelessly inadequate. But his own solution, mass action and equipotentiality, is scarcely a solution. It simply restates the problem. We are now in a position to look more deeply into the principles which make mental processes reliable in the face of unreliability or poor quality of components and data.

The major principle in, or perhaps even the overall description of, how the brain copes with an environment from which only fragmentary evidence can be obtained, and of how it copes with its own limitations and malfunctions, is that knowledge is embodied in the nervous system: knowledge both of the outer environment and of the characteristics of the system itself. It is not the case that brains are the only knowledge using systems. Indeed, it seems that a productive way of viewing the difference between the biological and the non-biological is precisely that living things are characterized by an adaptation to an environment, and that this adaptation consists of an embedding of knowledge relevant for survival about the environment and itself within the organism. Goodwin (1976), for instance, argues this case convincingly in the context of embryology.

Nevertheless, brains are particularly important instances of this capacity, because of the sophistication and complexity of their knowledge using processes. However, the reason why this cognitive, or knowledge using, process should not be thought of as confined to the brains of higher animals is that we can certainly see knowledge embodied in non-neural biological processes. It is this kind of knowledge which Chomsky (1965) refers to in his discussion of linguistic competence. Any native speaker has a knowledge of the grammar of her language: this can be reliably deduced from the fact that she can speak grammatically. But this knowledge is not separate from the processes of using the language. It is not the kind of knowledge that one would look up in a textbook or an encyclopedia, but knowledge embedded in the procedures of production or understanding linguistic utterances.

The knowledge in many biological processes is not separate from what the organism does with it. In an encyclopedia one can look up some item and acquire knowledge about it, but this requires that there be a process of gaining access to that information (reading), and then another process of deciding what, if anything, to do about it. Certainly in some circumstances we seem to be able to use and deploy symbolic entities in this rather disembodied, but flexible fashion. But more basically knowledge can be embodied directly within the process which makes use of it; embodied as part of the procedures for carrying out the organism's purposes in the world.

The two features which emerge from closed loop control systems described in chapter 5 on emergent properties illustrate this procedural embedding of knowledge. In the case of a regulator which is perhaps the simplest possible example, the relevant knowledge about the environment consists of a symbolic representation of a single scalar variable, which in the water balance system betokens a quantity such as cell volume or extracellular volume (see e.g. Oatley, 1973). Though this kind of symbolic instantiation is more often spoken of in terms of information, it seems better not to be mealy-mouthed, and speak about knowledge. A set point in a body fluid regulator is a genetically inherited piece of knowledge about the environmental conditions suitable for the life of body cells, and it is arranged in such a way that the knowledge actually takes part in the processes necessary for maintaining these conditions.

As land dwelling animals evolved, and the sustaining nutrient sea which had provided a benign environment for them was relinquished, they had to create a simulated sea within their own bodies: the extracellular fluids. And, as

Claude Bernard (1865) stated, the physiological condition for a free existence in a hostile environment is to maintain constancy in this stimulated sea, or, as he calls it 'internal environment'. What this means is that whereas the primordial sea, because of its mere size, had the effective qualities of constant temperature, pH, osmotic pressure, and concentration of various substances, not only does the genetic heritage of the organism need to contain the knowledge of these conditions, but the means for creating and sustaining them in the small volume of body fluid, which, if unregulated, would be subject to all kinds of insalubrious variation. It is the knowledge of the appropriate conditions for the environment of body cells, in control systems capable of maintaining these conditions in the face of hostile environmental perturbations that is embedded in the set points of physiological regulators.

Also in the system that controls water intake in mammals is knowledge of the limitations and characteristics of the physiological system itself. When an animal drinks in response to a fluid deficit, the water drunk does not immediately enter the body fluid pool, it suffers a delay of absorption from the gut. Hence, though the water has been drunk, it is not yet in the body fluids and cannot be detected by the body fluid receptors.

Thus an ancillary receptor system is arranged to monitor the amount of water flowing through the mouth and throat, and the distension of the stomach (see e.g. Oatley 1970). The signals from these receptors contribute to diminishing thirst by subtracting a signal of the amount drunk from the signals representing the fluid deficit and if they did not do so, the animal would go on drinking long after it had consumed sufficient water to repair its deficit. But the signal from the receptors in the mouth and throat cannot be permanently subtracted from the deficit signal which arises at the body fluid receptors, or else each time the animal got into water deficit and drank, the effective thirst signal on the next occasion would switch on only at a larger value of deficit. Rather the signal from the mouth and throat must decay at the same rate that water is actually absorbed into the blood stream. This rate of decay can be measured in experiments, and is indeed the embedded knowledge of the relevant absorption characteristics of the alimentary tract.

The other main property of the feedback control loop which

was discussed in chapter 5 on emergent properties, namely the property of non-linear oscillation, is again an instance of procedurally embedded knowledge, in this case of the periodic lighting sequence of the terrestrial environment. The models of this terrestrial rotation, which all circadian clocks comprise, are, again, not uncommited knowledge, but knowledge dedicated to creating the behaviour and physiology which fit the animal to the alternating cycle of light and darkness.

Thus, if an animal's adaptation to its environment includes a life strategy of relative advantage during the day, when it is light, like, for instance, most birds and primates, or if the animal is nocturnal like bats and rats, then an internal clock to schedule activity during the advantaged phase, and inactivity in a place of safety during the disadvantaged phase is clearly an important adjunct to adaptation. The clock model thus contains knowledge in the form of effective action to make for the adaptation. Animals are able to anticipate dawn, wake up, though they may be down a dark hole, remain quiet, still and unobtrusive during their disadvantaged phase. And all these things are without direct reference to the environment itself. For evidence from that environment is fragmentary: in this case often temporarily unavailable, e.g. if one is down a dark hole, or if one has one's eyes shut. Thus it is more reliable to behave with reference to an internalized model. And the model at the same time embodies the knowledge in the form of procedures generating behaviour appropriate to the knowledge it contains. It is such that it can accurately reflect the relevant properties of the environment. In the case of circadian clocks this includes the entrainment properties of circadian oscillators which keep them in time with the environmental cycle, and with each other.

These three processes of regulation, the overcoming of a delay in a feedback loop and the property of circadian oscillation illustrate three biological processes of knowledge embedding: to overcome the inherent unreliability of environmental inputs, imperfection of the biological system itself, and fragmentation of environmental data. Thus respectively, the structure of the regulator control system minimizes and compensates for what would otherwise be disastrous perturbations of the internal environment of the body fluids, namely, changes in concentration of solutes due to water loss which is bound to be suffered by land dwelling animals. The overcoming of the absorption delay in the feedback loop is a problem which engineers face continually in designing control systems, and is an inherent physical limitation of all control systems since it is typical that the time taken for a signal to be transmitted is a source of instability. The reference by animals with circadian rhythms to models of the rotation of the earth rather than directly to the environmental light pattern overcomes the problem of the temporary unavailability of the necessary data. It is typical of the problem of organisms' perceptual collection of data from the world, that this evidence is partial or even fragmentary.

Moreover, the regulator and oscillator processes just described also illustrate how embedding of knowledge of this kind, although it can and does occur in neural process can also occur in non-neural processes, because both regulation and circadian oscillation can and do occur in entirely biochemical systems.

Further development of the theme, into matters which are more specific to neural or similarly complex symbolic processes is best done in the field of perception.

IMAGE RECONSTRUCTION BY THE VISUAL SYSTEM

The first and simplest example I choose is that of image reconstruction by the more peripheral parts of the visual system. The human eye is a very imperfect optical instrument. The principal refracting surface is usually astigmatic, i.e. somewhat cylindrical in shape rather than circularly symmetrical, and this means that lines of different orientations in the environment cannot be brought into focus on the same flat or spherical surface. Often astigmatism is considerable in one or both eyes and requires the wearing of spectacles which are shaped to cancel out the asymmetry, or contact lenses which present a spherical refracting surface to the world. Then there is the pupil, which is small enough to bear comparison with the wavelengths of light and thus causes diffraction. The lens is not of high quality as lenses go, it is absorbent and a lot of light is reflected from its surfaces. Although its posterior surface is almost hyperbolic in shape, which reduces spherical aberrations, it does still suffer from these as well as a considerable amount of chromatic aberration. This latter means that light at the blue end of the spectrum is brought to focus well in front of the retina. Nature has done a bit of a bodge job on this problem, eliminating blue receptors from the fovea where acuity is most important, and interposing various yellow filters to attenuate short wavelength light. The vitreous humour is an absorbent medium, and apparently most absurd of all, there are the large blood vessels and several layers of cells in front of the photosensitive receptor surface. All these factors contribute blur in the retinal image.

The representation of choice in determining transmission characteristics of any optical system is that of Fourier analysis. The transmission function of an optical system can be characterized in terms of its response to spatial frequencies, just as the transmission function of an electronic or audio system can be characterized in terms of its frequency response for time varying signals.

Campbell and his co-workers, notably for instance Campbell and Green (1965) and Campbell and Robson (1968), undertook spatial frequency analysis of the human visual system by having observers adjust a contrast control of a sinusoidal grating displayed in oscilloscope screens to the level at which they could only just see the stripes of the grating. The reciprocals of the thresholds for sinusoidal gratings over a range of frequencies

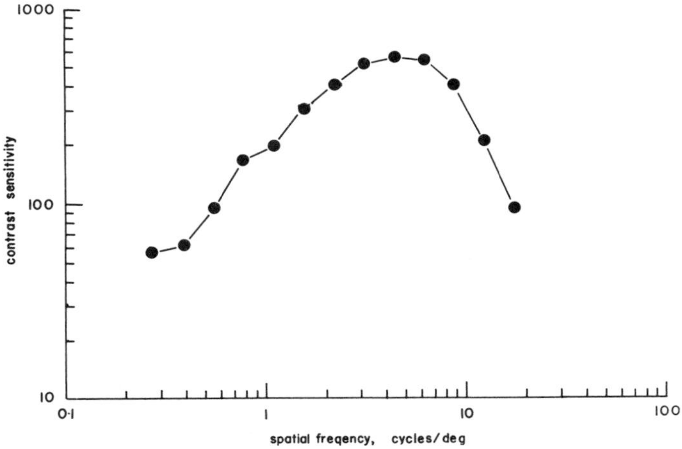

Figure 8.1 Contrast sensitivity function for a single human observer adjusting contrast to threshold level (from an experiment of P. Lennie; graph used by permission).

measured in this way were then plotted for form contrast sensitivity functions (see fig. 8.1).

One way to view the contrast sensitivity function is as the transmission characteristics of a rather low fidelity optical system. The progressive losses at higher frequencies are characteristic of any passive optical system. They describe in the spatial frequency domain the resolution of the instrument. In other words, for one reason or another any optical instrument will fail to resolve stripes at some frequency: the blur imposed by the instrument will merge them together. The high frequency attenuation is indeed the description in the frequency domain of the phenomenon of blur. This progressive attenuation of higher frequencies seen in the human contrast sensitivity function is not unusual in form, it is only unusual in comparison with other optical systems for the poorness of the response, i.e. the relatively low frequency at which the attenuation starts.

As described above, however, the eye is known anatomically to suffer from optical imperfections, and these together with the evidently low resolution power of the neural networks (perhaps reflected in the coarse receptor mosaic and the large receptive fields of retinal ganglion cells) are no doubt responsible for the form and position of the threshold function for human spatial frequency resolution. It is , however, important to note that this is a threshold function: the set of points at which signal is lost in noise, and is not necessarily characteristic of 'normal' human vision which we typically undertake well above threshold.

The decline in sensitivity of the human spatial frequency function at low frequencies is not characteristic of most passive optical systems. It reflects the fact that, as demonstrated by O'Brien (1958), we cannot register very gradual brightness gradients. Xerox copying has the same property. As discussed in the previous chapter, the effect is equivalent in the spatial domain to neural adaptation in the temporal domain. It is part of the visual system's admirable characteristic of being able to achieve adaptation to prevailing brightness levels locally, over each small area of the visual field, rather than globally over the whole field of view as is the case when selecting a film speed or an iris aperture in a camera. This local adaptation process in human vision is usually discussed under the heading 'dark adaptation' but is really a continual local adjustment to brightness levels on the retina. The receptor and other processes with a relatively small dynamic range of perhaps two or three log units (as suggested by, for instance, Werblin and Dowling's 1969 intracellular recordings from the retinae of mudpuppies) can operate positively and negatively about an average level for a small retinal area, as opposed to requiring an enormously larger dynamic range which would be required to operate about an average for the whole retina.

This local adaptation means, however, that overall brightness values are not detected directly by the human visual system, but extrapolated from what is taken to be happening at relatively well defined brightness boundaries. This is the significance of the O'Brien effect (O'Brien, 1958), in which a simulated pair of Mach bands will induce an apparent brightness difference between the two areas separated by this boundary, where there is no physical brightness difference.

The highly bowed curve of threshold contrasts for gratings, therefore, represents a transmission of very low fidelity. High and low frequencies are grossly attenuated compared with the peak responses at two to five cycles per degree. This threshold curve which is generated by the observer just being able to distinguish signal from noise then can be taken as a measure of the imperfections of the system. If, however, the way we saw was shaped by this filter characteristic, then no edges would be sharp, no brightness differences between non-adjacent areas of the visual field could be detected. Some textures, at about the frequency of lines of print in a book held at arm's length would seem contrasty, and all others finer and coarser would seem dim. In fact, we do not see like that, and the reason is that the brain is doing something about it. It is, indeed, another example of the classic Gestalt/Lashley problem of how the brain does cope with degenerate data.

The treating of the human visual system in Fourier terms is not just a frequency analysis of its transmission characteristic as one might analyse a camera. In the experimentation which used Fourier analysis there arose the suggestion from Campbell and Robson (1968) that the visual system itself might be undertaking some form of frequency analysis. The hypothesis was that the visual system contained independent channels each with its own threshold and each tuned to a particular spatial frequency. Campbell and Robson found that the threshold of a square wave grating (the Fourier components of which contain the fundamental frequency of the grating and its third, fifth, seventh and the series of odd-numbered harmonics) could be predicted from the independent threshold of its fundamental. This is in accord with the visual system itself making an analysis into frequency components. Moreover, they found that the point at which a square wave grating could be distinguished from a sinusoidal one was predicted from the threshold of a sinusoidal grating of three times the fundamental frequency. In other words, what primarily distinguishes a sinusoid from a square wave in Fourier terms, is the existence in the latter of a sine wave out of phase with the fundamental, at three times its frequency and one-third of its amplitude. Campbell and Robson claimed that at the point when this frequency would reach its independent threshold, as measured on the contrast sensitivity function, an observer was able to distinguish the square wave and sine wave gratings. Furthermore, Blakemore and Campbell (1969) had shown that adaptation to square wave gratings raised the threshold for sinusoids not only at the fundamental frequency, but also at the third harmonic.

Sullivan, Georgeson and Oatley (1972) also used an adaptation method; adapting observers to either a high or medium frequency grating, or to a narrow or medium width single stripe. Following adaptation, the observer's thresholds for sinusoidal gratings and for single stripes (bars) were measured. We found, as had Blakemore and Campbell, that adapting to a grating produced a frequency specific depression in the grating threshold function. However, adapting to a single bar did not produce a width specific depression in the bar threshold function. Rather the threshold for bars of all widths was raised. This is again in line with the notion that the visual system is undertaking some form of Fourier analysis. Single bars contain a wide spectrum of frequencies, and if thresholds for the stimuli used in this experiment depend on channels sensitive to particular frequencies, one would not expect any width specific adaptation, since a bar of any width would adapt a wide range of frequency channels. Furthermore, by the same argument, adapting to a bar of any width should depress the sensitivity to all gratings, and this is what we found. Moreover, adapting to a grating near the frequency of maximum sensitivity should depress the sensitivity to all bars, whereas adapting to a high frequency grating should have no effect on bars since this is a relatively insensitive channel and thus not important for threshold detection of wide spectrum stimuli. This too was found.

Since these experiments various pieces of simulation work, particularly that of McLeod and Rosenfeld (1974), have indicated that receptive field organizations of the conventional kind have frequency selective properties. Receptive fields such as those first described by Hubel and Wiesel (1959) in which a central elongated excitatory area is flanked by parallel inhibitory regions are spatial frequency filters.

The question then is this. Are the quasi-independent channels with properties of selectivity for spatial frequencies simply, as it were, accidental by-products of receptive fields organized for some other purpose and revealed only because Fourier analysis is a theory imposed on the system by experimentation? Or does frequency selection by the visual system itself perform some function in perception?

The probability is that frequency selection does have a real function. This is strongly suggested in a set of experiments by Georgeson and Sullivan (1975). They found that when observers were asked to match the contrast of different gratings above threshold to the contrast of standard gratings of fixed frequency and contrast, a set of curves was produced which did not follow the bowed shape of the threshold function. Rather, as the contrast of the standard grating rose, the equal contrast contours became flat. In other words, above threshold, the domain in which we typically undertake visual perception, our perception is not dominated by the very low fidelity characteristic indicated in the threshold function, rather it approaches high fidelity (in the frequency domain a flat response curve), and we see contrasts which are physically equal as perceptually equal right across the visible frequency range. This is, as Georgeson and Sullivan point out, another constancy phenomenon. Despite factors making for apparent inequality at the receptor surface, perceptual processes are arranged so that things which are physically equal in the outside world appear so to the observer.

The clue to explaining this contrast constancy phenomenon came from the computational deblurring of photographs taken from space vehicles, and other situations where the optical and other transmission characteristics of the picture-taking process exhibit a great deal of degradation. Using deblurring techniques, blur created by poor focusing, turbulence in the media through which the picture has been taken (and in the case of electron micrographs, aberrations) can be compensated for. The technique involves knowing or discovering the transfer function of the system in Fourier terms (Oatley, 1976). The picture is transformed into the spatial frequency domain, either optically, as in a hologram, or computationally. Then by applying an operation which is the reciprocal of the degradation transfer function, and inversely transforming the spectrum a reconstituted deblurred picture is obtained (see e.g. fig. 8.2). In principle the process is simple.

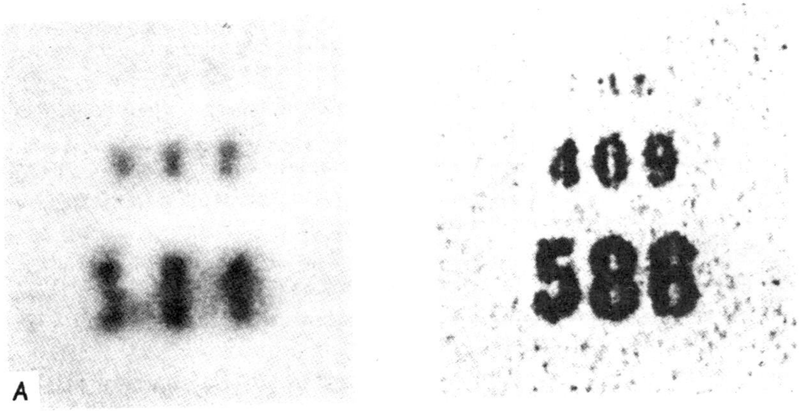

Figure 8.2 Fourier deblurring: on the left is a blurred original, on the right a deblurred picture produced by compensating in the Fourier domain for the original blurring process (from Gennery, 1973).

For instance, if a given spatial frequency is known to have suffered an attenuation, then its amplitude (contrast) must be multiplied by the reciprocal of that attenuation, and if it has suffered a phase shift, then that component must be shifted back.

Georgeson and Sullivan argued that this must be what the visual system is doing to create the flat, high fidelity, equal contrast contours from images which have suffered the considerable degradation known to exist in the eye. They argued that the bowed contrast sensitivity function only represents the situation at threshold, i.e. the points at which the signal is lost in noise. It does not, however, represent the sensitivity of the frequency selective channels throughout their range. If a given frequency can be detected at all in the retinal image, it seems to be multiplied by the reciprocal of its attenuation to provide an apparent supra-threshold contrast close to the physical contrast of the original pattern.

Supporting evidence for this idea comes from some further experiments reported by Georgeson and Sullivan in the same paper. Mitchell *et al* (1973) have shown that people suffering from astigmatism suffer a residual, evidently neural defect even after they have been wearing glasses for some time. With astigmatism, lines oriented in the same orientation as the astigmatism come to a focus at a different place than lines at right angles to that orientation. So accommodating to lines at one orientation automatically defocuses lines at right angles to them. Lines oblique to the astigmatism can never be properly focused. Mitchell *et al* found that even when optically corrected, astigmats showed markedly raised thresholds for orientations of gratings which were not aligned with their astigmatism. Presumably during the period of development the visual system, lacking sharply focused images in those orientations, had only developed to matching the low contrasts of those orientations. This may be related to the rather interesting recent controversy (see e.g. Barlow, 1975) as to whether animals lacking experience of contours in a particular orientation during a critical period of early life develop orientation sensitive cortical neurones in the normal way. Whether or not Mitchell's phenomenon is related to the neurophysiological findings, the neural deficit of threshold sensitivity of astigmats is well established, and Georgeson and Sullivan showed that this situation too was, in some astigmats at least, compensated above threshold. That is to say, that rather over half their astigmatic subjects set the contrasts of gratings above threshold and at different orientations, to equality when they were physically equal. This too seems explicable if the gain of frequency selective channels can be changed to compensate for attenuation of those frequencies by earlier parts of the system (e.g. by the astigmatism of the lens or the neural system).

The situation then seems to be this. The image in the retina suffers severe degradation due to a number of optical and neural factors. However, the visual system because of the organization of receptive fields is able to separate different spatial frequencies in the image into different channels. This process may be thought of as similar to making a Fourier transform of the image. The advantage of operating in this domain is that if the degradation characteristic of the system is known, it is a relatively simple matter to adjust the gain of each channel. So if a given frequency can be detected at all, it can be multiplied to compensate for its attenuation. The adjustment is very like adjusting the bass and treble controls of an audio hi-fi set to give a flat frequency response over the whole audible range. Whether any operation of phase shifting occurs is not known. Neither is it known what if anything corresponds to inversely transforming the spectrum back into the ordinary space domain.

The principle, however, is clear. This situation is of a classical kind: people can create an accurate perception of the outside world despite the fact that the immediate data on which the brain works is degenerate. The principle which Lashley did not fully grasp is that in order to do this the brain must have knowledge of the characteristics of the system, or the environment or more usually both.

In order to achieve frequency compensation, either of moon pictures or in the human visual system, the frequency response of the system must be known. In technological optics, this can be discovered by transmitting a known signal containing all frequencies in a known phase relationship, and analysing the response to this signal. The visual system might obtain this same knowledge by assuming that on average visual stimulation contains all frequencies at roughly equal amplitudes. Though the experiments of Mitchell *et al* on people's adjustments to wearing spectacles begins to address this problem, it is by no means solved.

There seem to be two ways of viewing this frequency compensation process. Either it can be seen as a preprocessing operation, perhaps set up in early life and staying relatively fixed, as suggested by Mitchell's results. Alternatively adjustments in the gain of channels could be made over periods of days, and certainly this would not be unexpected in view of results in experiments where subjects adapt to distorting prisms, some of the effects of which are to introduce aberrations (e.g. chromatic fringes) of the kind that the system already has to cope with. People wearing a new pair of spectacles also find that it takes a couple of days to get used to them.

Alternatively, it might be best not to think of this stage as a preprocessing one, but continually adjustable in the light of other operations in the visual system. The analysis of processes in the visual system not as a set of progressive immutable operations on data, but as a dynamic heterarchical set of mutally dependent operations is another principle of the brain's capacity to operate in the face of degenerate data and unreliability, and will be discussed further in this chapter.

The shortcoming of the idea that deblurring is a process which takes place at some particular peripheral part of the visual system, and then that the processed signal is passed on to the next stage is two-fold. First, in general it seems that perception at least sometimes requires the facility of returning to, and redescribing data processed nearer to the domain of the retinal image itself. In the previous chapter various preprocessing operations, a logarithmic transform of the digitized grey-scale data, and a lateral inhibition process were described in Roberts' (1965) program, but although these can be thought of as fixed preprocessing operations, so that their outputs are immutable in the light of further analysis, there might be circumstances in which it would be advantageous for the brain to adjust parameters over perhaps some part of the image, because of a high probability of the existence of some feature, not sufficiently clear to be detected using parameters set without *a priori* expectations.

FRAGMENTARINESS AND CONTEXT

Continuing the discussion of the previous chapter, we can recognize three modes of perceptual analysis. The most evident mode, and that assumed by many theorists, particularly physiologically oriented ones is a hierarchical scheme of 'bottom up' processing. Analysis starts at the bottom or lowest level, i.e. the retinal image, and proceeds upwards to 'higher levels'. The assumption is that an operation such as lateral inhibition might take place in the retina. The processed image is then passed on to the next higher stage for further processing and so on. The idea is quite compelling. It is indeed the idea of progressive stimulus classification. Physiology and anatomy seem to go hand in hand in this ascending hierarchy: the cortex is both anatomically and functionally higher in the hierarchy than the retina, and the lateral geniculate body is in between.

The second mode is top-down. It is also a hierarchical mode, and is the one in which Roberts' program mostly works, with cues in lower domains having the function (ideally) of identifying high level hypotheses or schemata which can then be applied to the data. Roberts' program has two stages of, as it were, blind bottom up processing, the logarithmic and the lateral inhibition transforms of the digitized image data, and then goes into top down mode, first to project lines, and then object schemata.

The third mode is an interactive combination of top-down, and bottom-up operations, usually called 'heterarchy'. I have argued that perception can hardly be thought of as perception without top down analysis, i.e. seeing retinal images as depicting things, means having cues in the image which point to what things, or higher domain entities, we might infer to be there in the outside world. But the overwhelming importance of context in perception, the fact that typically there are not 'stimuli' which have the same effect wherever and whenever they occur, but that any particular part of an image can be ambiguous, and is disambiguated by analysing the context in which it appears, implies not just top down analysis. It implies that (ideally at least) in some of the stages of analysis, the system can use whatever it happens to know including external context and its own expectations. Further, that as analysis proceeds, and some understanding of the meaning of the scene develops, this might modify the previously assumed interpretation, and thus it might be a good idea to return to reanalyse some lower domain descriptions in the light of this new context.

Although this issue of how far visual processing is bottom up (i.e. data driven) or top down (in terms of projected schemata) or heterarchical (with each stage able to influence each other) is by no means settled, it does seem from the recent work of Marr (1975, 1976) that data-driven preprocessing, up to the level of figure-ground separation might proceed autonomously. Marr calls the output of this analysis 'the primal sketch' and argues that this sketch is then 'read' by higher level processes. Though the way in which it is read will be influenced by the meanings which are to be attributed to it, computation of the primal sketch is not influenced by higher processes. This is in contrast to the heterarchical control structure of line finding described by Shirai (1975). If Marr is correct, then we can properly distinguish a set of preprocessing/line finding/figure ground segmenting operations from the more abstract schema projecting operations, just as they are distinguished in Roberts' (1965) program, with the construction first of a line drawing of the scene, which is then delivered to a further stage.

It seems then at the present stage of our knowledge that Marr's conclusion should probably be followed. This allows a set of operations, largely driven by data, although invoking the local schemata of lines and edges to be completed before object schemata are invoked. Following this though, more interactive heterarchical analysis is probably necessary.

One reason for accepting this conclusion is that perception is typically so quick as to seem instantaneous, and a completely heterarchical control would be slow. The speed of perception also argues that at the level of object schemata, understandings and expectations can be carried forward from moment to moment.

For this (and other reasons) Minsky (1977) has argued that many of our schemata consist of 'frames' or frameworks of knowledge which we carry around, and 'slot' new data or corrections into. Thus we have a great deal of knowledge about the construction of a 'normal' living room – walls, ceiling, floor, windows, door etc. so that we do not have to analyse the whole scene, rather we make corrections to the basic schema. Nor do we have to re-analyse a scene when we move around. Rather we carry forward the framework. This is the idea of 'schema and ocrrection' so compellingly argued by Gombrich (1960) in his famous book *Art and Illusion*. With Minsky's paper, although computational embodiment is not achieved, it may be that vision and language programs more explicitly exhibiting this principle are on the way.

In order to cope with problems of fragmentariness and damage, therefore, it seems that we need a structure which can carry forward, and project high level schemata, which has a rich understanding of context, and which can in addition 'try on' and revise various hypotheses, in a heterarchical fashion. Always it is advantageous to identify the most wide reaching, most meaningful hypotheses possible. After all, if you can see the cue of a nose, you not only know that there is a person in the scene but where to look for the eyes, and the body, and so on.

Though perception typically seems instantaneous, it can be slowed down so that we can experience and perhaps make conscious some of the kinds of knowledge-using processes which typically occur in unconscious inference. One way is to use a deliberately fragmentary figure, and pay attention to our thought processes while trying to make sense of it. Here, for instance, is a fairly well known picture, which is often quite difficult to see at first.

Look at fig. 8.3, and for those who find it difficult to see 'as' something meaningful I will give some pieces of context, both

Figure 8.3 The hidden man (from Porter, 1954).

of overall setting and specific details. I will use here the description of Abercrombie (1960) from her excellent book on the schemata of perception and judgment. Looking at the picture at first we usually get

> the information that there is a meaningless patchwork of black and white blotches. The messages from the patchwork on the retina can, however, be interpreted in another way, as the head and shoulders of a man. Some people think the picture resembles a medieval representation of Christ. His face is turned towards you, and occupies the middle third of the upper half of the picture. The top of the picture cuts across the brow so that the top of the head is not shown. The face is lit from the observer's right hand side, so that the eyes are in shadow and the cheeks and chin brilliantly illuminated. His hair and beard are long, but the chin is clean shaven and is a white spot catching the light just above [and

a little to the right of] the middle of the picture. A white cloth covers the right shoulder and slopes across the breast – the left shoulder is turned a little away from you and the right upper sleeve is a black area in the lower left part of the picture.

The picture may appear as suddenly as when a light is switched on. Some people cannot see it with the help of words only, but need someone to trace the outline of the features over the patchwork. The object has not changed, nor has its image in the retina, yet the information received from the object is different – no longer is it seen as a chaotic patchwork but as the picture of a man, sharp clear and characteristic.

If that figure still cannot be seen, then turn the page and look at a shaded outline drawing (fig. 8.4) incomplete in a different way and then re-inspect the figure. Different people, no doubt because they have different 'person schemata' or stereotypes, find different examples of these kinds of figures hard or easy to see. Amongst other things, what can happen with such figures is that one can get hooked on a particular hypothesis about part or all of the figure, and be unable to stop seeing that particular interpretation. We can get stuck in a hypothesis, which is difficult to dig ourselves out of. But it is usually possible to, eventually. We can create the new theory, arrive at a better representation, a more meaningful perception. But it is this kind of partial hypothesis, which fails to make sense of the whole, which we often seem to keep getting caught up in, in all our thought patterns, and which makes some kind of heterarchical, re-analysis, and at a more fundamental level, reprogramming, necessary to perceiving and learning.

To give a more structured account, a computational metaphor, of seeing processes I will now briefly discuss two programs, one by Clowes (1971) which demonstrates the contextual diasambiguation of ambiguous picture segments, by a knowledge of three dimensional geometry of opaque polyhedra. The other by Falk (1972) shows further the operation of cues and schemata, and a structure of theory of the picture taking process, being used to attack degenerate, fragmentary pictures.

If we take any line drawing of a scene containing opaque plane-sided polyhedra, that is to say, line drawings of the kind that could conceivably be delivered at the end of the first set of stages of Roberts' (1965) program, one of the features we might notice in the picture domain are junctions, that is to say, the meetings of two or more straight lines at angles to each other.

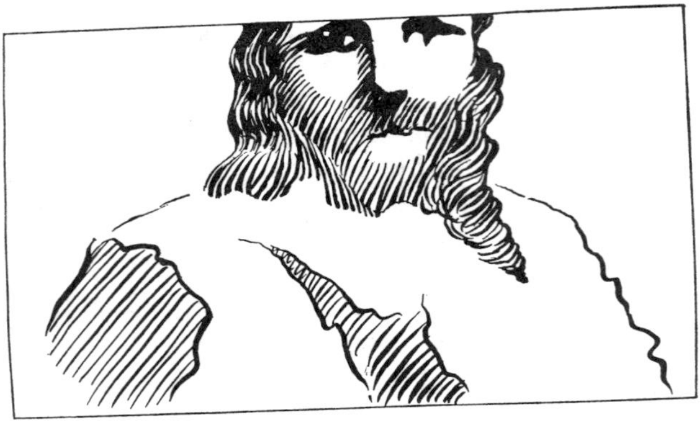

Figure 8.4 The hidden man revealed (from Abercrombie, 1960).

Guzman (1969) was the first to give an account of such junctions and some of the uses to which they could be put. Guzman's discovery was that one could assign junctions to a relatively small set of categories, (see fig. 8.5) and that each type provided more or less strong evidence that the surfaces depicted as lying between the lines of the junction, did or did not meet at the edges depicted by the lines. At a T junction (as was pointed out by Helmholtz) the likely interpretation is that the two surfaces on either side of the stem of the T meet at an edge depicted by that stem, whereas the third surface at this junction, the other side of the cross piece of the T, is likely to be a surface of a nearer object, partly obscuring the surfaces which join at the edge depicted by the stem. The inference is that the crosspiece is the edge of a nearer surface which in the 3-D world does not join the other two surfaces. Guzman treated other kinds of junctions as well. These are shown in fig. 8.5, and he gave each one an intuitively appealing interpretation as to the strength of evidence that each line in a junction was or was not an edge joining two surfaces represented by the two adjacent regions in the picture. (Notice here how it is important all the time to keep separate the descriptive terms used in two different domains, cf. table 1 (ch. 7). Thus line, junction and region are descriptions in the domain of line drawings, whereas edge, corner, surface are in a domain of 3-D scenes. The task is to interpret a description in terms of

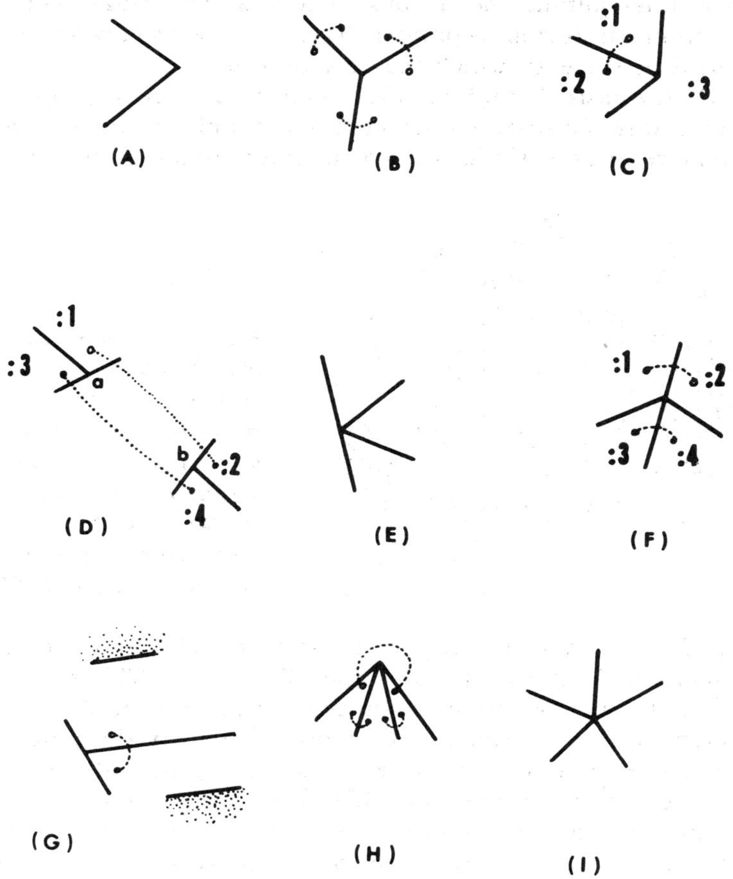

Figure 8.5 Junction types used by Guzman. For each type of junction, whether the configuration will be treated as evidence that adjacent regions are part of the same 3-dimensional body is indicated by a link. Links are shown here as dots joined by curved dotted line. Thus junction type b (FORK) is taken as evidence that all 3 regions meeting at the junction are parts of the same object, whereas for type c (ARROW) regions 1 and 2 are joined, but both are separate from region 3, (from Guzman, 1969).

one domain, i.e. the line drawing, in terms of some description in terms of another domain, e.g. a description of the objects and their disposition in the scene.)

The junction types then seen in fig. 8.5 are labelled with little links joining the regions, if in that particular type of junction the regions separated by a line are usually surfaces joined by the edge which that line depicts.

On the basis of weighing this evidence, in a not very sophisticated way, Guzman constructed a series of programs which would return descriptions of which regions of a picture such as

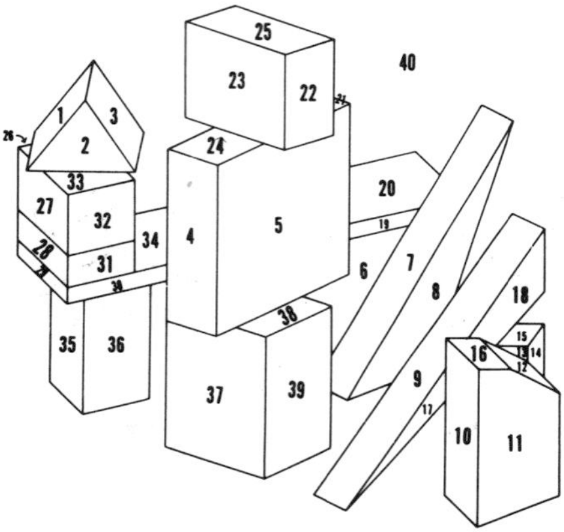

Figure 8.6 A picture which can be successfully segmented into groups of regions corresponding to the 3-dimensional bodies in the scene by Guzman's program, (from Guzman, 1969).

fig. 8.6 belonged together as surfaces of each discrete three-dimensional object in that scene. Winston (1972) gives an account of the evolution of Guzman's programs, and how the weights of various kinds of evidence offered by the junction types were modified, with Guzman also including rules to take into account the context of other adjacent junctions.

Guzman's analysis is rather incomplete, however. It offers no account of the disposition of the objects or surfaces in space. Merely it lists which surfaces belong together on separate 3-D objects. It is a kind of figure-ground segmentation. In order to take the analysis further, a more sophisticated analysis of context, and a more explicit theory of how disposition of plane-sided opaque polyhedra could generate types of junction in a line drawing was needed. Both Clowes (1971) and Huffman (1971) conducted such an analysis independently, and I shall here follow Clowes' version.

Clowes first restricted the class of plane-sided polyhedra that could appear in a scene to exclude any object in which more than three surfaces met at a corner. In fact, as Clowes points out, at each corner of a typical plane polyhedron, exactly three surfaces meet. Clowes is also much more explicit than Guzman about the descriptive significance of domains. So he describes the picture domain in terms of lines and regions, and also their relationships in four types of junction: ELL, ARROW, FORK and TEE.

He then defines the scene domain as an organization of polyhedral entities. The entities of interest are edges, surfaces and corners, and the significant relationships which these entities can have are that two surfaces may join at an edge which may either be convex as where one looks at the edge of a brick, or concave, as when one looks at the inside of a box. Convex and concave edges are, as it were, intrinsic to the object, and independent of the viewpoint. But there is another feature of an edge which is dependent on the viewpoint. A line in a picture may separate two regions which do not join at the edge depicted by the line. That is to say, a surface may obscure another surface which cannot be seen from the viewpoint. In this case the line indicates that one of the regions depicts a surface which is not joined to, but is wholly or partly behind, the other. The effect can be seen if one puts a matchbox on a table in front of one. Then the edge of the box farthest from the viewpoint indicates an unseen surface of the box, obscured by the top surface of the box. And the edge in question indicates that the surface of the table, and the seen surface of the box do not meet at that edge.

By construction of a lot of polyhedral scenes with glue and cardboard Clowes discovered a kind of geometry, or ecology of the blocks world which would be embedded into the procedures of a program to make sense of line drawings of that world. For instance, in the domain of three-dimensional polyhedra there are intrinsically just four types of corner at which three surfaces meet. These corner types depend on how many of the three edges that join there are convex (the remainder being concave). Thus a type I corner has three convex edges, a type II corner two, a type III one, and a type IV corner none (i.e. it has all concave edges like the inside corner of a box). Furthermore, from a particular viewpoint there may be 0, 1, 2, or 3 surfaces of any corner visible. Thus in the scenes domain including intrinsic and viewpoint dependent elements there are 16 corner types, and fig. 8.7 from Clowes' paper illustrates some of these, with the Roman numerals being the corner types and the Arabic subscripts the number of surfaces visible from the viewpoint of the picture.

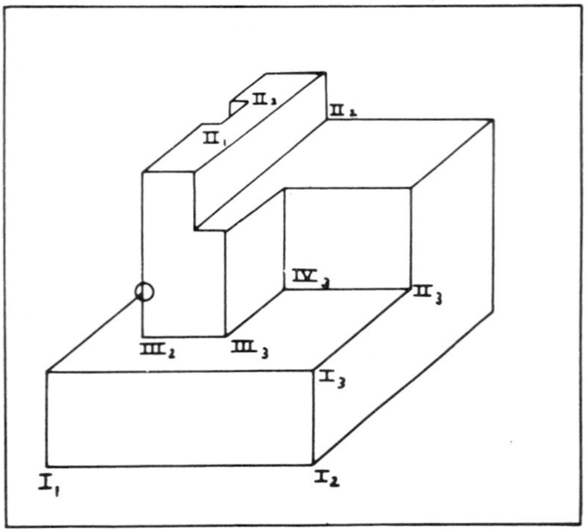

Figure 8.7 Picture of a 3-dimensional object with the different kinds of visible corner designated by Roman numerals, with the subscripts indicating how many surfaces are visible at that corner. Notice how the same corner type, e.g. type I, can be depicted in the picture by different junctions: e.g. here type I corners are seen depicted by ELL, ARROW, and FORK junctions, (from Clowes, 1971).

The task that Clowes set himself was to design a program which would produce an interpretation of a line drawing in terms of the entities and relationships (corner and edge types) of his scenes domain.

I will not give details of the program here, but merely say that it works by choosing one junction in the picture, listing its possible interpretations in the scenes domain, and then moving to adjacent junctions and doing likewise. The program uses the context of adjacent junctions to disambiguate the multiple ambiguous interpretations. Thus a line of development might start with supposing a particular fork junction to be composed of all convex edges, at a corner where all edges are visible. This clearly labels the lines emanating from that junction. Hence an interpretation deriving from the next junction which labelled one of those lines as being a concave edge, or an edge with one surface invisible, would clearly be incompatible with the interpretation of that edge derived from the first corner.

Going around a set of junctions in a picture and comparing interpretations allows the program to search for a set of mutually compatible interpretations for the whole scene. For a legitimate plane-sided polyhedron picture (in which the objects have no holes) this program will come up with at least one interpretation. Interestingly it may also come up with more than one possible interpretation. Thus the program (rightly) delivers several compatible sets of junction/corner cum line/edge interpretations for the picture shown in fig. 8.8. There

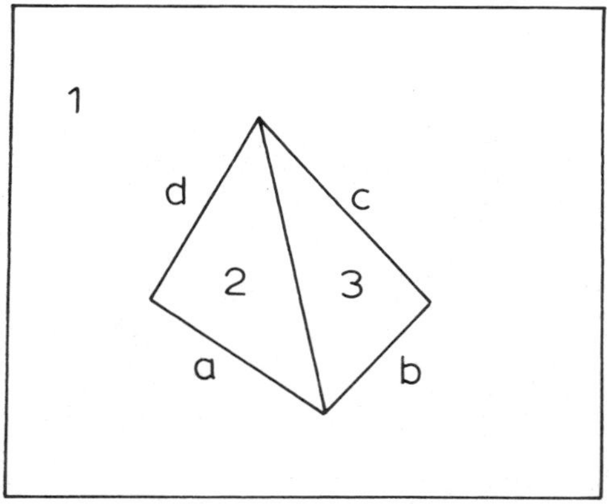

Figure 8.8 Picture of an ambiguous scene, see text (relabelled after Clowes, 1971).

are three visible surfaces here (labelled 1, 2, 3) and amongst other things the scene might be a tetrahedron resting on a surface (1), with only two of its four sides being visible (2 and 3). Ambiguously it could be resting so that lines a and b represent the edges (concave) at which the tetrahedron meets the base surface (1) with c and d being lines depicting convex edges with a hidden surface behind them, and the corner at which they join being up in the air. Or c and d could be on the ground surface and a and b in the air. There are other interpretations too. And from another viewpoint the picture composition of this scene could be quite different e.g. with three surfaces of the tetrahedron being visible. But in this case the basic meaning of the scene, i.e. a tetrahedron on a base surface, would be the same.

Clowes emphasizes that his approach is a linguistic one. In

other words, the scene itself has a semantics or meaning: the nature and disposition of the blocks relative to a viewpoint. As in linguistics there can be ambiguities, which in ordinary perception tend not to occur because we resolve them using a lot of contextual knowledge. There can be paraphrases, e.g. the same scene from different viewpoints, and yielding quite different surface structures in the picture domain. Moreover, there can be anomalies, failure to produce either syntactically or semantically well formed structures. Clowes program works on the basis of eliminating these anomalous, badly formed structures in which, for instance, according to the geometry of the blocks world, a line cannot represent at one end a convex edge and at the other a concave one. Indeed, the program is able to reject as an 'impossible object' scenes such as that shown in fig. 8.9 for which there is no mutually compatible set

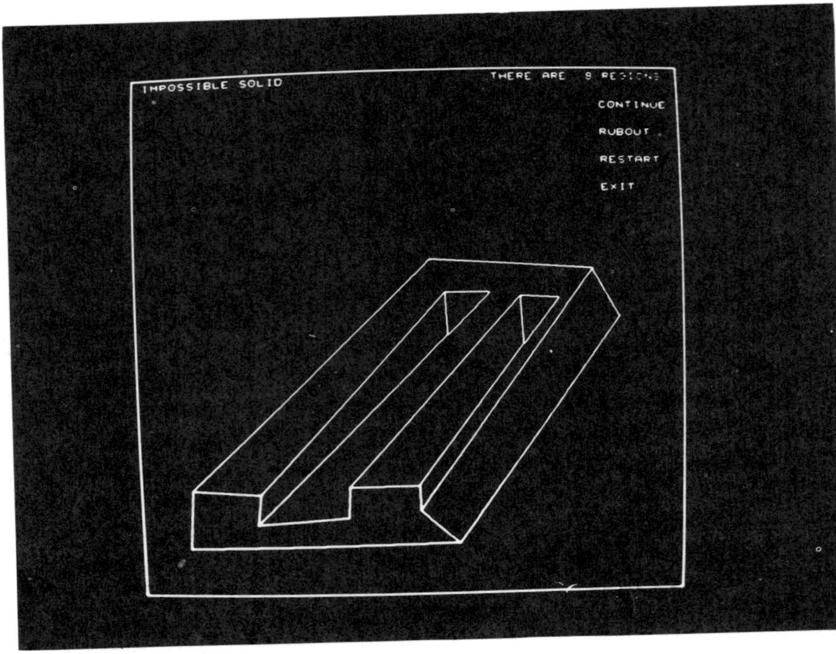

***Figure 8.9** Photograph of visual display of computer running Clowes' (1971) program. The program can find no mutually compatible set of 3-D interpretations of the junctions here, and therefore describes the scene as an 'impossible solid', (from Oatley, 1972).*

of interpretations of the lines as convex, concave, and hidden surface edges.

PROCEDURALLY EMBEDDED KNOWLEDGE

The linguistic analysis can be carried further by juxtaposing what is perhaps the best known artificial intelligence program by Winograd (1971) with a scene analysis program by Falk (1972). Winograd has shown how in order to make sense of a sentence a letter string must be parsed syntactically, and the interpretations continually referred both to a structure of general knowledge about the blocks world (e.g. that blocks can be stacked on top of one another) and specific knowledge about the current layout of the scene. This knowledge is represented in the computer in procedures which specify what to do about the states of affairs that can arise. Procedures also point to other procedures which contain alternative routes, if one happens to be impossible because of the general or specific state of the blocks world.

All the time while trying to make sense of a sentence, the program uses whatever it knows in a highly interactive way. Thus, if the parser after operating its lexical and syntactic procedures delivers the notion that the string of symbols, 'the red block', is a candidate for a noun phrase, and the logical subject for a sentence, the program will check to see if there are such 'red blocks' in its world, and also what the reference for the determiner 'the' might be. Clearly 'the' must indicate some specific red block; presumably either the only one in the scene or one that has been mentioned before in the conversation. Thus the effort after meaning proceeds with the program using whatever it knows from its lexicon, from its representation of grammar, from its general knowledge of the blocks world, from the specific current state of the program's representation of that world, and from its memory of the conversation that has taken place previously. It uses any and all of this knowledge, whenever and wherever appropriate, in a flexible control structure which can invoke the different types of knowledge whenever they seem as if they might be appropriate. It is this kind of structure which is known as heterarchical as opposed to the more rigidly hierarchical, unidirectional processing modes of bottom-up and top-down.

Moreover, the knowledge is embedded in procedures in the form of what, linguistically or in term of action in the blocks world, the program should do about the various interpretations that arise.

Following Winograd's program, and despite its shortcomings (of which there are many) it appears that a plausible conversation partner, or language user, could scarcely operate other than by using a great deal of general and specific, linguistic and non-linguistic knowledge in a very flexible, even opportunist, fashion.

It seems, moreover, that to perceive one must again deploy and utilize knowledge and inferential processes in some similar fashion. This in part is what Falk's (1972) program sets out to do.

Falk's program is in a sense an extension of both Roberts' and Guzman's. This is to say, it is designed to accept a photograph of a blocks world scene, and like Roberts' program it has prototypes for the objects which will appear in the scene, and it attempts to use information from the picture domain to identify those prototypes, and then project 2-D constructions of its prototypes back on to the picture. In the process, Falk uses Guzman-type junction heuristics to segment the picture into sets which are candidates for the separate objects in the scene. What is new in Falk is that, unlike Roberts, the program is tolerant of missing lines, not recovered from the photograph because of bad lighting, shadows etc, and the program uses knowledge of the structure of domains higher than the domain of picture points in order to reconstruct the missing lines, of the fragmentary image. Also new in Falk is that he articulates and deploys a theory of support: how blocks can be supported by the table and by other blocks.

In short, the program relies principally on the following kinds of procedurally embedded knowledge. First, there is an explicit theory of the picture taking process, the projection of a three-dimensional scene onto a two-dimensional surface given a particular viewpoint. Secondly, the program knows the three-dimensional position of the camera relative to the table on which the blocks are placed. Thirdly, the program's prototypes are of nine solids of fixed size, of which it knows the 3-D structure and dimensions. Apart from the line finding part of the program (which from Falk's account may or may not have been implemented), the program also knows (fourthly) both

Guzman type segmentation techniques, and how to extend these to reconstruct lines that seem to be missing from the picture. Fifthly, the program has a theory of support of blocks by the table, and of blocks by other blocks. Finally, although the program is most of the time straining to get into top-down mode and project its prototypes onto the picture, if the 2-D structure derived from the projection of prototypes (the program's hypothesis) does not produce an adequate match with the original picture, then the program will return and try to re-interpret parts of the picture domain data.

I will not describe here the workings of this rather complex program in detail. Apart from Falk's own paper, there is an excellent account of this program in Sutherland (1975). Here I will merely try to give some flavour of how Falk tackles the problem of degenerate line data: a degeneracy which is bound to occur in any real image producing process and is occasioned principally by shadows and changes of brightness on the surfaces of objects, changes which can in the domain of picture points be much more substantial than the variation of brightness across a picture segment depicting a three-dimensional edge. And as fig. 7 by Clowes (1973) shows, it is entirely possible to 'see' the existence of edges which do not appear as brightness gradients in the picture at all.

As the figure from Falk's paper (fig. 8.10) shows, the program is faced with two kinds of reconstruction task. First, there is, as shown in fig. 8.10a, the set of lines missing because they have not been recovered by the line finding part of the program. Secondly, there are the notional missing lines which arise as the program succeeds in dissociating picture segments belonging to separate blocks in the scene. These are the lines which, from a particular viewpoint, are hidden behind opaque bodies, and this is a problem already attacked by Roberts using his program's knowledge of the projection of prototypes.

In fact, Falk tackles this problem by defining some junction types as degenerate versions of other junction types. Typical is the case of fig. 8.10a in which there are four ELL junctions, i.e. junctions at which only two lines meet, which plausibly could be incomplete three-line junctions, created because of an under-enthusiastic line finder. Falk tries to identify such incomplete junctions. Some of these should 'really' be TEE junctions, and thus be cues for segmentation of an obscuring from a partly obscured body, though they can also arise from

3-D corners and hence should be assigned to other junction types; e.g. in fig. 8.10a one of the incomplete junctions 'should be' of type ARROW. However, in the segmentation problem

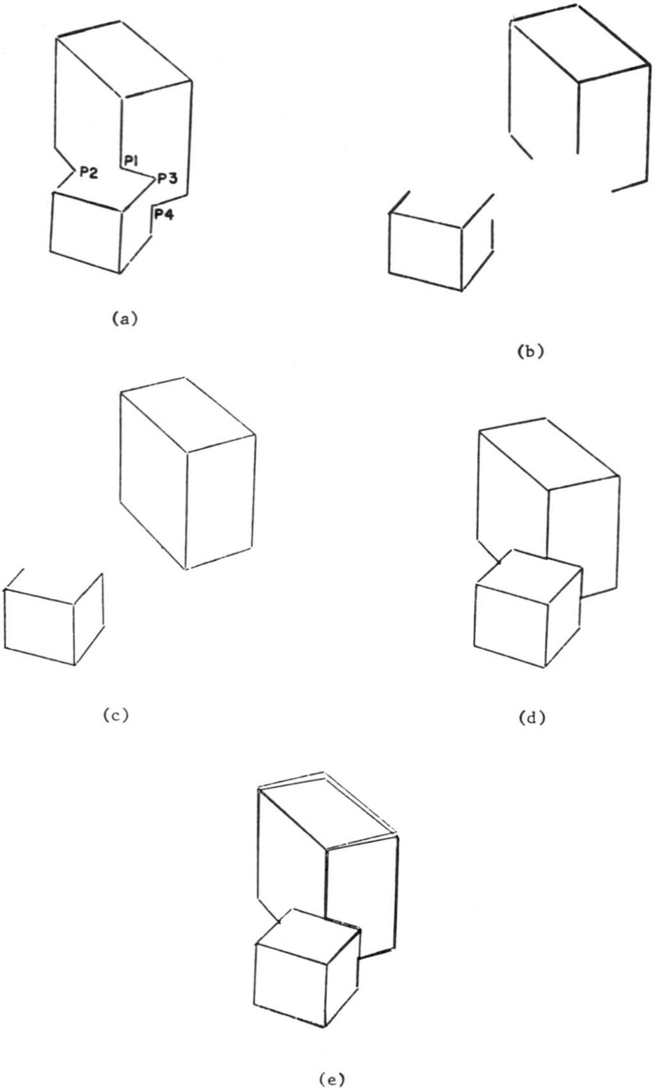

Figure 8.10 Stages in Falk's program, see text for explanation, (from Falk, 1972).

Falk is concerned mainly with degenerate TEE junctions, as cues to segmentation. So an inference is constructed that a vertex can be assigned to the class ELL if it makes an angle of more than 180 degrees with the background (e.g. like the top-most junction in the picture of fig. 8.10a, or when both the lines meeting at the junction are also lines in the cross strokes of adjacent TEE junctions (as for instance the upper ELL junction of the smaller block in fig. 8.10d. Otherwise the junction is labelled BAD ELL, and the knowledge of what to do about that is embedded in a procedure which assigns lines joining at the BAD ELL vertex to separate bodies. It is largely the operation of this heuristic which produces the segmentation seen as one passes from fig. 8.10a to fig. 8.10b.

Following segmentation, line completion techniques of a fairly obvious kind are applied within the segmented bodies: e.g. joining of co-linear line segments, extension of lines with free ends to meet at a junction. In this kind of way the structure of fig. 8.10c can be produced, and by this stage Falk is essentially into the same kind of process as that followed by Roberts of using cues in the now 'separate' pictures of bodies to invoke appropriate prototypes. The projection of these onto the picture will allow further line/edge reconstruction of lines 'lost' in the picture taking process, edges obscured by intervening bodies, and edges obscured behind the body in question.

Apart from the backtracking which Falk's program will undertake if the final 2-D projection of his constructed scene does not provide a good fit with the original picture data, Falk makes less use than he might of heterarchical transfer of control in the program. But the program structure is rich enough to make the implementation of such processes possible, i.e. knowledge available within the working program could be used at various stages to disambiguate various uncertain interpretations at various points.

There are some vision programs which work within a more explicitly heterarchical structure than Falk's. Winston (1972) gives a tentative set of guidelines for heterarchical control which has been developed at MIT.

1 Procedures should embody knowledge and try to accomplish something (a goal). Moreover the system should try to get wherever possible into a top-down mode — seeing descriptions in lower domains as something at a higher level.

2 The executive control should be distributed throughout

the system, so that modules and procedures interact not like a master and slave, but like a community of co-operating experts.

3 Programmers should make as few assumptions as possible about the state of the system in which a procedure will be called i.e. about where some piece of knowledge and what to do about it could be useful.

There is now, moreover, a growing collection of vision programs each of which probes a little further into making explicit the articulation of knowledge which would make seeing a pictorial 2-D image as a scene possible. This is not the place to review this work; there are, moreover, recent reviews of these programs (Winston, 1975; Mackworth, 1976; Raphael, 1976). Most of the programs are still in the blocks world, though even here the articulation of knowledge which is required, for instance, to allow shadows in a scene (e.g. Waltz, 1975) become quite involved. Shadows in real photographs make for a lot of difficulties with much more substantial loss of line data from the picture domain. But, on the other hand, in three-dimensional interpretation they also make the task easier by allowing entry into a whole new branch of theory about the structure of the seen world, since shadows imply a light source positioned apart from the observer's eye. Thus theoretically one can determine the position of the light source (which will be co-linear with the shadow boundaries and the edges that cast them) and then one effectively has two viewpoints of the same scene, an enormous help to seeing the world as extended in three-dimensional space. (This is, of course, the underlying significance of shadow cues to depth in human vision, as well as stereopsis and motion parallax.)

Beyond the blocks world, of course, we have the world of our everyday perception of our environment, where more and more contextual knowledge, not just of three-dimensional geometry, and the theory of lighting and viewpoint, is brought to bear, still in the processes of unconscious inference. There is knowledge of how things are constructed, culturally dependent knowledge of how to live in urban or rural environments, knowledge of causality, of people and animals and their repertoire of actions, and our expectations, and desires in all these regards.

One of the few excursions into this domain, and, furthermore, one which very explicitly deploys the idea of perception being the effort after meaning by the projection of aspects of our cognitive schemata on to the data is by Weir (1975). Her program tackles the problem of making sense of kinetic displays inducing the perception of causality which were first investigated by Michotte (1963).

There is a large variety of interpretations which subjects make of the kinetic display of two dots approaching one another and then moving in various ways subsequently. These include pushing, triggering, striking, passing, carrying away, frightening off etc. The movements can be seen in various circumstances as animate or inanimate, and both physical causality (as, for instance, in an interaction like shove half-pennies) and psychological causality like chasing away can be attributed. The animate interactions can be seen as motivated and purposeful, with attributes such as friendly, or hostile. Weir's program makes such interpretations on the basis of various cues (attributes of the frame-by-frame movement sequence). Various 'readings' of the situation arise because of the different modes and speeds of interaction and the necessities of 'explaining' new positions which are not predicted by the preceding sequence.

The program does not (in one sense) add to Falk's treatment of how whole scenes in the object domain can be constructed from fragmentary data, but in another sense it shows how an inferential structure can make contact with a yet further domain of actions, intentions and causes, where attributions are inherently ambiguous, and the data on which they are based are in some sense less 'complete' than in line drawings of the blocks world. After all, when we 'see' a causal interaction what 'happens' is a spatial and temporal conjunction of events. We supply the cause, or the motive, from our schemata. When we enter this domain we begin to inhabit the world of common sense, where, for instance, a mark on paper is seen as having resulted from the movement of a pen and the person performing this action of writing is seen as having intentions.

We are still some way from being able to offer satisfying metaphors of the interpretations we make of our own and others actions in the world, and of the results of matches and mismatches which occur when we project our schemata into the social domain. Weir's program moves in this direction and this is surely one which should be followed.

LASHLEY REVISITED

Although Lashley identified the problem of reliability of function despite degenerate data, multiple surface manifestations of the same object (as in different viewpoints) and the damage of the system itself, it is clear that he was not himself able to offer any very convincing suggestions. Curiously in a seminal paper on motivation (1938) he argues against a generalist notion: 'I suspect that all cases of motivation will turn out to be ... not a general drive or libido ... but the partial activation of a very specific sensory motor mechanism'. In his theoretical statements about vision, however, and his ideas of mass action, he seems to be generalist in the extreme, i.e. he seems to be arguing that a generalized structure can in some context-free manner transform the co-ordinates of the visual field into the co-ordinates of movements and actions.

What Lashley seems to have been missing is any way to get hold of and supply productive metaphors for the representation of knowledge, and the effort after meaning. In the experiments of Artificial Intelligence we find that specific knowledge must be represented in ways that make possible the achievement of specific goals. And the problem of fragmentariness is not addressed by the creation of some generalized machine with transforms input into a structure like Lashley's (1942) diffraction patterns, or the Gestaltists cortical field forces, or Cowan's statistical neurodynamics, in which the particularities of the retinal image, and its imperfections and fragmentariness somehow go away leaving the underlying significant generalities. Although some such general strategy as a transform or filtering operation can be very useful in preprocessing, the main structure has to be rather specific to the tasks of the organism in its particular environment, and to the aspects about which it will form theories. Though specific this structure must be flexible and capable of being an interpretive and active representation of the world with which it relates.

In the account I have given, the apparent differences between the problems of so-called stimulus generalization (in which a single object may be recognized despite differences of retinal size, or position or viewpoint), and motor generalization, and fragmentariness of the data which impinge on the receptors, and the resistance in the brain to loss or damage or malfunction of its parts, become one. Thus the structure which can cope with an image which has parts missing or which has poor definition is also one which can cope with differences in viewpoint which display or obscure different features of a scene. The system has enough flexibility to construct an interpretation of a fragmented image because it has many heuristics, and many interacting routes to the same goal, and much knowledge (or 3-D geometry, projection, lighting, causes, actions etc) which can be brought to bear on the same problem of interpretation from different directions. It is clear without further argument that such a system would also function despite malfunctions or damage of its own internal parts.

SOME IMPLICATIONS FOR PSYCHOLOGY AND PHYSIOLOGY

I do not want to say a great deal more about the implications of all this for the methodology and theory which is deployed in psychology to address the problems of mental processes and behaviour. I hope I have already said enough to indicate some of the difficulties under which our current 'textbook' approaches are labouring.

It is clear that as far as psychology is concerned, we are no longer restricted to an experimental method which has to define stimuli, create experimental environments free of the rich contexts in which people normally operate, and to try to isolate 'the mechanism' by which a subject performs this or that task. Such methodologies can be (though they are not always) trivializing. Worse, they seem before the outset of the experiment to contain a strong commitment to the view that there are isolatable pieces of behaviour (responses) and isolatable causes of that behaviour (stimuli). It also seems to imply that if we isolate and understand the parts, it is a simple matter to put these parts conceptually together to make a whole. If the brain is interactive and dependent on context; context which is moreover ever changing, and often unrecognized by experimenters (e.g. the social pressure of white coats and laboratories) then trying to strip away context, and trying to avoid interactive effects can be trivializing and self defeating.

Just as linguistics offered another route to the mind, via Chomsky's (1965) exposition of how paraphrase, ambiguity and anomaly can be used to expose the linguistic competence of the language user, computation offers another route. It is the route of being able to experiment with systems that represent and use knowledge, in an interactive way. It is the route which instead of trying to take a biological mechanism apart tries to construct one which will address the same problems of perception or language or whatever, which people address. In so doing it seems one can discover or invent some of the principles that make mental processes possible. It is a route which instead of trying to strip down context, and creating only an alien environment, can try and work towards the interpretation of context-rich environments of real conversations or real visual scenes.

For physiology some of the same conclusions hold. But, in addition, if the mental processes are founded on heterarchical principles, or principles of cues and schemata, and can operate despite fragmentariness or damage, this puts some conclusions drawn from the recording from the single nerve cell, or the attempt to relate by ablation or stimulation some particular piece of behaviour to a particular part of the brain in a very questionable position. Particular parts of the brain may take part in the generation of a sequence of behaviour in some circumstances, although they may not be strictly necessary for that behaviour. There seem to be many routes to behavioural goals: it is the interacting structure as a whole, rather than its individual parts which are important.

9 *Perception and theory in science*

Perception can be characterized as making meaningful sense of data collected from the outside world. Typically data offered to us in visual and language form are incomplete. The problem is to take these fragmentary ambiguous data and interpret them so that we can understand the world in terms of our relationships with it. The argument developed in this book has been that in order to do this successfully the perceiver must bring to bear representations of knowledge. Also it is probably not coincidental that this is exactly the problem of the scientist. He or she also is faced with scattered and incomplete data, of varying reliability, and (amongst other things) the choice of directing attention to these observations or those. The task is to make sense of the data, and this is done by applying a theory. A theory is more or less adequate for the purpose the scientist has in mind. It is essentially a schematic representation of knowledge which articulates some observations in a particular way, and rejects others as irrelevant. It is an abstraction which allows us to make certain kinds of inferences easily, to understand certain aspects of the universe within the terms of particular purposes we might have in that universe.

The operation of schemata within perceivers' minds involves the projection onto the data of their theories of the way the world is, and seems to be controlled (not always tightly) by cues of various kinds, which the visual system can compute from the retinal image, as well as a knowledge of the general setting or context in which the perceptual act is taking place. In this sense perception seems not very different from the operation of prejudice. A man exhibiting a cue such as a black skin, or long uncombed hair, or a bowler hat, will allow us to project onto its exhibitor a great deal of knowledge (or rather beliefs) about who that person is, what he is like, whether or not we might want to talk to him or even whether we would feel happy about his marrying our sister. It is implausible for anyone to claim to be free of prejudice. But, of course, we can use more or less evidence to cue our perceptions.

Science, too, is a belief system operating rather like other belief systems. It is not necessarily, in practice at least, a 'rational' or a privileged view of the world. It is a set of theories about the world which allow us to see it in certain ways. Its implicit purposes are those of predicting, explaining and controlling certain aspects of the world. As a representation enabling those kinds of tasks to be accomplished it seems quite good. Rockets have been landed on the moon, effects of different agricultural methods have been assessed, weather can be forecast and bacterial infections can be arrested, all with varying degrees of success according to the adequacy of current technology and of the current representations we have of the phenomena in question. At the same time as scientific representations seem quite good for some purposes, they seem fairly unhelpful for others: understanding certain kinds of experience for instance, or conducting personal relationships.

There is, of course, one sense in which science does claim to be a privileged view of the world, and this is the sense argued eloquently by Popper (e.g. 1963). The mark of a scientific, as opposed to a pseudo-scientific statement or theory, is in its testability, the possibility of its refutation by some observation. Thus, statements in physics, such as that bodies of unequal weights fall at the same rate in a vacuum, is testable. Statements derived from psychoanalytic theory, such as that slips and accidents are motivated by the unconscious, cannot be refuted. Though there may be many instances in which the idea may seem to be confirmed, it is less clear that there are observations that could disconfirm the idea. Popper is careful to point out that this does not mean that psychoanalytic or other statements of a kind which he calls mythological are not meaningful, or insightful. Simply, he argues that they must be demarcated from those theories which could be potentially refuted, that is to say, critically tested. Scientific theories then apply to aspects of the universe which are isolatable, stationary and repetitive. In those circumstances by processes of conjecture and refutation, we can make successive approximations to, though not attain, descriptions of the universe which within their own terms are true. This, of course, puts psychology, where phenomena are not typically isolatable, stationary or repetitive, in a difficult position.

Perhaps the question to ask about any theory particularly in psychology is not whether it is true, but how well it makes meaningful sense of a range of phenomena of interest within the terms of purposes we might have for them: is the representation an effective one, is the model or metaphor or theory apposite? Although it is clear that it is of first importance for a theory to have some strong reference to an external reality, as well as to judgments of internal consistency, tests of the theory, or its refutability, are by no means always crucial to its value.

In the history of psychology it is possible to exhume any number of experiments from journals, e.g. some of those testing the Hullian drive-reduction hypothesis (Hull, 1951), which would be largely without interest if published today. This is not necessarily because the issues they were concerned with have been resolved; it is not even that Hull's theory has been found to be 'false' (though many arguments have been advanced against it). It is simply that the concerns of psychology are no longer what they were in the fifties. Hull's theory, and the experiments surrounding it seem now to many psychologists irrelevant. Thus the question is not whether Hull's theory was true or false. Rather it may simply seem pointless.

It is not always clear what the aims and purposes of psychology really are: evidently not the disinterested pursuit of knowledge, not entirely to promote human wellbeing. The difficulty is that without some understanding of purposes and aims it is difficult to see how well a particular representation of knowledge is adequate to meeting those purposes. Some individual psychologists' motivations (e.g. desire for personal recognition, see Hagstrom, 1965) may be hinted at but the aims of psychology in general sometimes seem more elusive, and maybe that is why psychology seems to be particularly susceptible to fashions.

But a fashion is only an unkind term for a small-scale version of what Kuhn (1962) called a paradigm. A paradigm can be thought of in one way as what appears in a current textbook in any particular discipline. It might be useful to distinguish three levels of paradigm in psychology. First there is the lower level paradigm, or fashion. At the time of writing the dominant paradigm in academic psychology can be characterized as the 'information processing approach', and a typical text is Lindsay and Norman's *Human Information Processing* (1972). At the next higher level I have been arguing in this book that a great deal of psychology and brain research is carried out within the framework of a paradigm which originated with Descartes, and which focuses on stimuli, responses and the connections (physiological or logical) between them. Acting as a third level umbrella paradigm experimental psychology and brain research embrace the notion of Science. Although Kuhn's analysis was of paradigms as existing within science, the analysis can be extended to see science as a paradigm in itself.

The first chapter of many textbooks of experimental or physiological psychology are about psychology as a science. Here for instance, in his *Foundations of Physiological Psychology* (1967) is Thompson: ' "mind" and "consciousness" have no measurable properties and hence cannot be defined in measurable terms ... The important point is not really whether terms like "consciousness" refer to something "real", but rather what kinds of phenomena can be measured and hence studied scientifically.'

Thus often the study of psychology, including physiological psychology, becomes defined as 'scientific', and this in turn allows some things to be included (e.g. behaviour) and other things to be excluded (e.g. conscious experience). As Kuhn (1962) has pointed out, this paradigmatic aspect of science has the effect of 'defining for the individual scientist both the problems available for pursuit, and the nature of acceptable solutions to them.' Furthermore as Merton (1942) has indicated, scientific procedures have acquired the status of moral imperatives. Thus procedures are not just adhered to because they are efficient (though they may also be that, and the justification for them may be in such terms), but because they are felt to be right and good. Merton identifies the transcendance of national and other sectarian barriers, the sharing of scientific knowledge among the scientific community, personal distinterestedness, and organized scepticism as the dominant mores, or moral imperatives of scientists. All these are high-minded ideals.

In this notion of psychology being a scientific pursuit there can be seen a strong restatement of what Bartlett (1932) said about cognitive schemata. Schemata are characterized both by a general frame of reference, and by an attitude. Paradigms in other words are the theories, or cognitive schemata that scientists use to make sense of their professional world. Like other schemata they are representations which articulate some observations and reject others; and the effectiveness of the representation differs for different problems. The practice of science is a metaphor for the operation of schemata. Putting it another way, trying to make sense of the fragmentary observations in scientific periodicals and of one's own experimental results is very like a scene analysis program trying to make sense of a photograph.

Just as Roberts' program (1965, discussed in chapter 7) looks for line segments, and tries to see configurations of picture points as lines, so a scientist looks for the repeatable and the measurable. It is not simply that he or she ignores other events, but within scientific theory (just as in Roberts' program) there is no means at all for seeing events other than those articulated by theory. Similarly, just as the program tries to see the scene as an arrangement of 3-D objects about which it knows the characteristics the scientist tries to see observable events as arising from some mechanism or process for which he or she has an explanation, i.e. a structure of inference.

Some authors, e.g. Abelson (1973), talk in terms of belief systems as involving the interposition of oversimplified symbol manipulations between the holders of beliefs and the real world. However, if it makes sense to talk of anyone having a belief system, then we all have at least one, and as I have been arguing here science is a belief system, is a paradigm, is a cognitive schema, is a representation which allows us to make sense of the world in a particular way. I, as a conscious being, may be able (as Bartlett, 1932, suggested) to turn round on my cognitive schemata, but I cannot step outside them. In a recursive fashion, what I write about the influence of paradigms or belief systems on psychology also refers to what I write.

Despite, or because of, this I now intend to argue that there are other goals and purposes beside explanation, prediction and control which people might have, and that, furthermore, the dominant psychological paradigm of stimuli and response imposes an even smaller and more restrictive peephole than necessary through which to view psychology.

EXPLANATION, PREDICTION AND CONTROL

Although it is possible to see scientific activity as a disinterested pursuit of truth, by a process of successive modification of testable theories, there also seems no doubt that the area in which this process works best is that in which events can be predicted and controlled. One may indeed wonder, in that case, whether the purposes of science are those of prediction and control of the world. We are not surprised to find that much of the subject matter consists of explanations, that is to say, descriptions in terms of causality or dependency or probability. In other words, explanations are precisely those kinds of model or representation that cast a problem into terms of prediction and control. So pervasive is the 'scientific' way of looking at things that for many it is difficult to imagine any other way of conceiving the world. However, there have been other structures of belief in European thought; there still are other belief systems in various parts of the world. In order to get the flavour of a belief system devoted to different ends and purposes, one way is to choose, and try and immerse oneself in the structure of some school of thought from ancient times, or another culture. Thus, for instance, the expression of thoughts and ideas in the medieval or the Renaissance world view is quite different from our own (e.g. Yates, 1964). To give a brief example: the angels in medieval and early Renaissance thought clearly have many roles. One of them is the expression of hierarchy; so there is an order of angels which from highest to lowest is Seraphim, Cherubim, Thrones, Dominions, Virtues, Powers, Principalities, Archangels and Angels. Hierarchies can express the idea that people and things have a place in the universe. They express the distance and relationship of people and things to the Divine, routes to take on spiritual journeys, or the routes of influence from the heavens to the earth. The hierarchy of angels also seems to express what is important in that belief system. For instance, the activities of the highest orders of angels were to speculate or contemplate on God.

Clearly where contemplation of the Divine was an activity of the most important of angels, it would be seen to be of high importance for people too. And if this is taken as a purpose, then the representation of knowledge or the cognitive schemata needed for this might be very different from schemata dedicated to purposes of explanation, prediction and control. Thus rather than standing at a 'scientific' viewpoint and labelling other belief systems as primitive, as naive, as silly, or demonstrably false, we could regard them as representations of knowledge as more or less suited to particular purposes and activities (which we might or might not share). A representation such as the Cabbalistic tree, or some of the structures of medieval and Renaissance thought might not be much use for designing a nuclear power station, or understanding some property of fundamental particles, but, on the other hand, the belief systems of physics and engineering might not be much use for such medieval concerns as, for instance, taking a spiritual journey, or indeed more modern preoccupations, such as conducting one's personal relationships.

The point that I wish to make here is that psychology can be conducted within a scientific belief system, and this is indeed the dominant form of contemporary psychology. But although this has the admirable quality of referring theories to externally testable reality, it also seems to have led to restrictions of a certain kind. Scientific psychology becomes a psychology of prediction and control; a psychology of explanation and causation. It does not necessarily provide a good representation for acquiring insight into one's own mental states (as opposed to explanations of them), and it does not necessarily provide a basis for conducting human relationships. It is probably no accident that even social psychology which is dedicated to understanding how people behave in social interactions has become highly manipulative both in form and content: a paradigmatic example being Milgram's (e.g. 1974) studies on obedience to authority in which subjects are hoodwinked into believing that they are administering painful electric shocks to people who are actually accomplices of the experimenter.

I move now from the paradigm of science in general to what I have characterized as the dominant paradigm within psychology, which is that of identifying patterns in the environment, patterns of response to those stimuli, and the lawful or causal connections between stimuli and responses.

It can be seriously doubted whether this characterization of psychology can live up to its own expectations and purposes, given what we have already found out about the brain.

If, in the view expounded here, the brain is well characterized by being able to operate with very incomplete information, and constantly projects its own knowledge onto the world, then we might seek a psychology of cognitive schemata being addressed by cues and signs (see e.g. Barthes, 1972; Goffman, 1974), but scarcely a psychology of stimuli. We might well have a psychology of flexible and creative representations of events and problems or of the attribution of meaning, but scarcely a psychology of connections between stimuli and responses. We might well have a psychology of how purposes are achieved, but scarcely one of responses.

The emphasis on repeatability and experiment in science is thus not simply a prescription allowing falsification, and hence critical testing, although operations such as the experiment avoid attribution of causal status to events which have no causal significance. Repeatability also powerfully expresses the purpose of prediction and control. For if one is to predict, it is important that events are repeated on all identifiable occasions, or at least are known to occur with a particular probability. It is important that individual instances are not unique. Similarly, if one is to control, it is important that setting up a series of prior events will produce a predicted outcome, on each occasion required, and when the manipulation is practised with appropriate objects. Statistics used in psychological experiments are an expression of the need to see subjects in experiments or surveys as similar and repetitious, individual variation (in this context) being dismissed (i.e. because it is not handled by the theory or schema) as chance variation, or experimental error.

But if mental processes are characterized by creative variation, by the generation of new representations in efforts after meaning, then perhaps we need not always emphasize repeatability. If even in experiments where the subject's task is trivial but apparently still subject to changes in the subject's strategies, then perhaps experiment does not of itself provide a guarantee of achieving adequate and true descriptions.

Kuhn (1962) has remarked of a scientist working within a paradigm that he 'usually seems to know, before the research project is even well under way, all but the most intimate details of the result which that project will achieve. If the result is quickly forthcoming, well and good. If not, he will struggle with his apparatus and with his equations until, if at all possible, they yield results which conform with the sort of pattern which he has foreseen from the start.' In other words, he scientist is operating with a schema which is primed to attribute meaning to some events, and to reject or ignore others.

The experiment then, although with its emphasis on isolating the causal variable, is also a device for specifying the kind of outcome that could be recognized as a valid outcome.

Furthermore, the manoeuvre of keeping all conditions but one constant, whilst varying the condition which is a candidate for causal significance, does indeed allow one to isolate single causes where they are isolatable. But it also has the effect of studying these causal candidates one (or at most a few) at a time. It has the effect of recommending extraordinarily impoverished environments for experimental subjects to operate in: the Skinner box, the darkened room with the subject staring at a spot of light and pressing a small switch.

But if perception is ordinarily highly dependent on context, then stripping away context may be a strategy of doubtful value. If mental processes are highly interactive, then the isolation of causal events, and their investigation one by one, may lead to a trivialization of psychology. Hoping that one can somehow combine a whole set of component processes and understand how a whole interactive system works may be an example of the reductionist fallacy.

Psychology may today be at the threshold of a paradigm shift, a crisis, and indeed this may be true for science in general. The view offered to us by science and technology invites us to see ourselves in a relationship with our world which is one of manipulation and control. Weizenbaum (1976) in a remarkably cogent critique of just the kinds of computational advances that I have been describing in this book makes the case against accepting science's offer of power over the environment. 'Science offered man power. But, as so often happens when people are seduced by promise of power, the price exacted in advance and all along the path, and the price actually paid, is servitude and impotence.' The computer, argues Weizenbaum, is just the latest in a series of implements which radically affect the way people see themselves in relation to the world. He gives a picture of the computer bum, denizen of the world's computing laboratories who seems to have formed some kind of symbiotic relationship with the machine. 'Bright young men of dishevelled appearance, often with sunken glowing eyes, can be seen sitting at computer consoles, their arms tensed and waiting to fire their fingers, already poised to strike, at the buttons and keys on which their attention seems to be as riveted as a gambler's on the rolling dice.' Computation, argues Weizenbaum, offers a universe which can be entirely controlled. Thus the will to control can become compulsively realized.

One aspect of this which Weizenbaum argues is that in this sense the computer is not so much unique as representative of the way in which technology offers new and potentially dehumanizing relationships with the world. A second point is that in so far as computation is a new departure we should not use it as a substitute for our human concerns, or believe it to be the vehicle by which all our problems in psychology, for instance, are solved. To do so is to adopt an immodest claim for final mastery over the sorts of issues which in their very nature computation as such cannot be appropriate for.

The view I have taken in this book is that computation offers a repertoire of metaphors which have many advantages over the metaphors drawn from the more familiar furniture of the physical world. With that I hope Weizenbaum would agree. What computation, or any other product of science or technology is not, is a method either of explaining away human mentality, or superseding it.

One of the troubles with the controlling manipulative view of the world which can inadvertently be derived from science is that it has within it a quality of alienation. We come to see ourselves as being apart from a world which we control. We can come to see other people too as things to be manipulated and we can see ourselves as things also to be acted upon. Clearly these are not the only relationships we could have in the universe. Other people in other cultures have seen themselves as being a part of the universe, taking part in the ebb and flow of its events, and in an earlier European culture people felt themselves not to be able to manipulate the world as such, but to have a particular place in a structure which included the universe and their fellow human beings. What seems lacking in our present culture is a sense of wholeness of the person, and of the person's relationships with the world. Rather, aloneness, fragmentation, compartmentalization and alienation seem ubiquitous. Moreover, the manipulative controlling view of the world in some situations leads to self contradiction; as in: 'If I had a slave whom I could command to love me on pain of death, her love could only be an unsatisfying sham, because I would have commanded it, and love is only love if freely and spontaneously given.'

In some sense this problem is well expressed by the difficulties surrounding the dichotomy between personal experience on the one hand and the theory of an objective world of causation and mechanism on the other. And this dichotomy is itself illustrated in the realm of psychology by Laing (1967)

> Personal action can either open out possibilities of enriched experience or it can shut off possibilities. Personal action is either predominantly validating, confirming, encouraging, supportive, enhancing, or it is invalidating, disconforming, discouraging, undermining and constricting. It can be creative or destructive.
>
> In a world where the normal condition is one of alienation, most personal action must be destructive both of one's own experience and of that of the other. I shall outline here some of the ways this can be done. I leave the reader to consider from his own experience how pervasive these kinds of actions are.
>
> Under the heading of 'defence mechanisms', psychoanalysis describes a number of ways in which a person becomes alienated from himself. For example, repression, denial, splitting, projection, introjection. These 'mechanisms' are often described in psychoanalytic terms as themselves 'unconscious', that is the person himself appears to be unaware that he is doing this to himself. Even when a person develops sufficient insight to see that 'splitting', for example, is going on, he usually experiences this splitting as indeed a mechanism, so to say an impersonal process which has taken over, which he can observe but cannot control or stop.
>
> There is some phenomenological validity in referring to such 'defences' by the term 'mechanism'. But we must not stop there. They have this mechanical quality, because the person as he experiences himself is dissociated from them. He appears to himself and to others to suffer from them. They seem to be processes he undergoes, and as such he experiences himself as a patient, with a particular psychopathology.
>
> But this is so only from the perspective [perceptual schema] of his own alienated experience. As he becomes dealienated he is able first of all to become aware of them, if he has not already done so, and then to take the second, even more crucial, step of progressively realizing that these are things he does or has done to himself. Process becomes converted back to praxis, the patient becomes an agent.

One of Laing's achievements is to realize and expound the idea that repression and suchlike, which Freud studied as processes and mechanisms, can better be thought of as modes of experience. For to experience oneself as mechanism, or as split into part mechanism, to experience oneself as alienated, not human, not whole.

And so one debate within psychology is in some sense about whether to concentrate on experience or mechanism. The resolution of this, however, is not in terms of one or the other: a representation in terms of mechanism or in terms of personal experience. The differences among different schools (e.g. experimental versus humanistic psychology) are themselves symptoms of this alienation. And what seems to be needed are representations of mind which will begin to accomplish some de-alienation, some joining of or at least statement of vital relationship between the two poles. And we as psychologists must ponder whether our activities in prompting images of man which are almost wholly images of mechanism are not contributing to the alienation that makes for people's experience of themselves as being split, repressed, mechanistic, controlled, or in some other way alienated, both internally and with their fellows and their world.

Though one can sneer at, for instance, alchemists from a perspective of modern chemistry, they seemed at least to avoid some of the dehumanization which some of us find in 'doing science'. For the chemical activities were externalizations, metaphors for the inner experiments and search for the philosopher's stone. And not only were the external processes thought not to be possible without some inner personal progress, but the inner progress was thought to be assisted and informed by the externalized metaphors.

It seems possible at least that we are now in a position to make certainly not the same de-alienation that the alchemists were seeking, but one more in tune with both modern science and modern experience. The new paradigm, moreover, for psychology at least seems to be shaping around the issue of meaning – the issue to which I have tried to address myself in this book.

Let me give two examples of schemata which seem to approach some de-alienation of the disjunction between objective science and mechanism on one hand, and personal experience on the other.

One of them is Kelly's (1955) theory of personality and personal constructs. Kelly expounds a theory of personality based on the idea of 'man the scientist'. In other words, he deploys the metaphor used earlier in this chapter, that the problem that people face is roughly the problem of making meaningful sense, within the terms of their own theories of themselves and their world, of the data that arise from interactions with persons and things in the world. Here then is a formulation in which the externalized, and rather formal activity of 'doing science' is used as a mirror to the much more personal and universal process of 'living life', and the indications seem to be that there is some helpful, de-alienating, mutual cross fertilization in Kelly's formulation.

In this context it is interesting that Popper (1963), the strong advocate of scientific procedure as a means for approaching truth, at least in the sense that potentially refutable theories assert something about reality, himself offers the metaphor of the unscientific, uncritical mind, not only as the basis of neurosis, but as the basis for various 'unpleasant' forms of authoritarianism in society.

> Psycho-analysts assert that neurotics and others interpret the world in accordance with a personal set pattern which is not easily given up, and which can be traced back to early childhood. A pattern or scheme which was adopted very early in life is maintained throughout, and every new experience is interpreted in terms of it: verifying it, as it were, and contributing to its regidity. This is a description of what I have called the dogmatic attitude, as distinct from the critical attitude, which shares with the dogmatic attitude the quick adoption of a scheme of expectations — a myth, perhaps, or a conjecture or a hypothesis — but which is ready to modify it, to correct it, and even to give it up. I am inclined to suggest that most neuroses may be due to a partially arrested development of the critical attitude ... to resistance to demands for the modification and adjustment of certain schematic interpretations and responses'

The metaphysic that Popper is espousing is that we only really learn by our mistakes (refutations). As we apply our schemata to the world by living, they fail in various ways and we can learn, change and develop by modifying our schemata or theories accordingly. Popper quotes J.A. Wheeler at the beginning of his book as saying 'The whole problem is to make the mistakes as fast as possible...'

The second, though less well known example I shall give is the movement towards what I will call 'convivial computing'. It includes the LOGO project of Papert and his colleagues (e.g. Papert, 1973). There is also the gradual diversion of attention in artificial intelligence from simply 'making models of intelligence' such as robots (though as I have aruged in this book, this activity has been valuable) towards a more complete appreciation, study and involvement in the interaction between the computer and the world, the computer program and the programmer, and the programmer and the world with which his or her program interacts (e.g. Papert, 1973; Goldstein, 1974; Hewitt, 1971). Also it includes the production of both cheaper hardware and software which will make computing in a mode of the procedural representation of knowledge more widely available and transparent to all kinds of people from school age upwards, in systems which react, and with which people can interact in a variety of creative modes.

The best way to explain these rather recently burgeoning developments is by reference to Papert's LOGO project. In this project children around the age of ten and upwards are given access to a teletype or visual display unit which is connected to a PDP-11 computer. This in turn is connected to a number of peripheral devices, for instance, to a toy vehicle called a turtle which the child can program to move around, and leave an ink trace so that it can draw patterns and pictures, to a video display on which static or movie pictures can be produced, to a music box on which music can be synthesized, and indeed to any other kinds of device with or without 'sense organs' which will interact with the environment or the programmer in whatever way one can imagine.

There are a number of what Papert calls 'powerful ideas' embodied in this project, and amongst them are the following. What we need to do in education argues Papert is to give people both better things to do than the typical rather passive sitting behind desks, and better ways of thinking about what they are doing. Sitting behind desks and 'absorbing' knowledge from a 'teacher' may well be an apposite form of socialization into a hierarchical and mildly authoritatian culture, but it may not be as good as it might be for allowing people to take responsibility for themselves in a spontaneous and creative fashion. Thus, rather than having syllabuses, which people must digest, and then at a later time regurgitate (the alimentary metaphor of education), an alternative arises of giving people an additional creative medium which is moreover in some ways more powerful and flexible than other creative media, and in which a person may pursue a project of his or her choosing.

In the prosecution of such a project, typically involving writing a program to do something like compose a tune, make a movie or write poetry, the person not only is operating under his or her own motivations, but can interact with a system which tests his or her designs and aspirations against a real environment. There is in other words in the writing of a program to do something, the development of a theory about how to do it, the externalization of the theory in symbolic form in the program (a kind of essay capable of being executed in a real environment), and a progressive interaction between the externalized theory, the environment, and the person externalizing the theory. In this way the programmer creates successive approximations and modifications of the process that the theory is designed to generate. Again we have the metaphor of the scientist and the developing theory, or schema, of the environment with which he or she interacts. But now the metaphor is in a more dynamic form. In part the dynamism comes from both the power of computation and the possibility of relatively rapid learning from the 'mistakes' that the program/programmer makes.

Although we do have the adage that we only learn from our own mistakes, most educational process denies this in important ways. People do not necessarily have very much that is their 'own' in educational processes. The methods, the form and the content of educational practice are more typically chosen for them. Interactions with this environment may allow people to learn, amongst other things, how to abdicate responsibility for their own education to someone who 'knows better', and that it is important not to be seen to 'fail' (see e.g. Holt, 1969). Children indeed learn a large number of creative ways of playing the system so that they do not make fools of themselves, though some of these ways can also be fairly destructive of the person, e.g. 'I never was any good at French' (despite the fact that the person speaks his/her native English perfectly) or a retreat from what are seen as 'intellectual' pursuits. Educational practice thus tends to create an environment in which the worst possible thing to do is to make a mistake, and, therefore, a fool of oneself. A not uncommon reaction is to switch off altogether so as not to lay oneself open to this personally damaging label of failure.

In contrast, though successive attempts at programs by children do produce frustration when the program fails to execute what they had in mind, they tend to feel not 'I am a failure', but 'It (the program) has a bug in it' (went wrong), and then to set about debugging their program, and hence their own theory of what they want to do.

This metaphor of learning how to debug one's programs, to debug one's theories, and how to debug one's own thought processes is perhaps the most promising line of activity to emerge educationally from this project. Typically it is not true that a person who learns to operate creatively in a particular medium, e.g. painting or mathematics thereby transfers the learning from his or her own mistakes in this medium, to other aspects of life. It is indeed not known whether this transfer and generalization arises from interacting with one's own programs in a LOGO project, but because the project allows and indeed encourages both doing and thinking about what one is doing, and because too a metatheory of bugs (mistakes) and how they arise, and how they might be tackled develops alongside the specific projects, the situation looks hopeful.

It seems at least possible that some of the reasons why people are so afraid of making mistakes, so reluctant to recognize them and hence learn from them (but rather prefer to avoid or repress them) have to do with our alienating educational process. Activities like the LOGO project may start to initiate an improvement. Here at least the mistake (the experiment in trying to succeed in a person's own aspiration) is usually presented back to the programmer when he or she runs the program, and in general this can be perceived as an invitation to improve, modify or abandon the theory or schema which generated it. Maybe that kind of attitude would make it easier to recognize our own neuroses and contradictions (mistakes).

Another of the 'powerful ideas' in this kind of computation is the offering of an alternative to experimental science as a route to understanding natural processes. Typically the scientist's solution to the problem of how to find out about something is to conduct an experiment to isolate the causal factors. The computational alternative (expressed in artificial intelligence and in the LOGO project) is that if you want to understand something about seeing or conversing, or walking or whatever, then you attempt to construct a computational device which will carry out whichever of these activities you choose. In so doing you will find yourself having to try and solve the same set of problems which the brain has had to solve in accomplishing these tasks, and thus having to discover and/or create the principles on which cognitive processes can be founded. Armed with this repertoire of metaphors we may be in a better position to examine biological instances of cognition. Furthermore, the creation of a process which perceives or converses or whatever has the de-alienating effect of relating mechanism to experience in that it is the programmer's own experience with the progressive debugging of his or her own theories which creates the development of these theories which are schemata, which are understandings of the principles underlying perception, linguistic conversation or whatever.

At one end of the spectrum this kind of process gives rise to the 'eureka' experience of a little girl in the LOGO project, using a phrase structure grammar to generate sentences, and exclaiming 'Oh, now I see why they have nouns and verbs.' At the other end of the spectrum is the more 'professional work on vision by academics' some of which has been described in the previous two chapters, and which has led to new departures in understanding the principles underlying perception.

What one sees perhaps rather distantly on the horizon is an era of more convivial computation in which the availability of cheap hardware, of a cost somewhere between that of a television and a motor car, and the development of transparent software, in which knowledge can be embodied in procedures about how to carry out sub-tasks in the projects one might conceive, might lift 'the computer' from the present status of the rather sinister, expensive, carefully guarded and sequestered calculating, controlling and data processing machine, into that of a creative medium. Though some seeds seem to be present they may take some time to grow, and computation may either become institutionalized or be seen (like mathematics) as too difficult or too specialized except for a small elite, so that the hopeful signs may prove to be chimeras.

There are weaknesses and pitfalls in the deployment of the computational metaphor in psychology and physiology. Some of them have been pointed out by Weizenbaum (1976). There are others. Although computational metaphors for psychological processes are testable against the reality of seeing whether the program will run successfully (a criterion a great deal more stringent than that met by most psychological theories) it is not clear that they meet Popper's definition of testable theories. But then if the human mind really is as creative and flexible as it seems to be, then it is not clear whether any theories of mentality would in the nature of things meet that criterion.

Even as ways of thinking about mind which may be productive, computational metaphors still labour under many difficulties. For a metaphor to be productive its recipient must be able to bring the relevant experience to the data to which the metaphor refers. Not many people have this experience of computation and maybe this will always be the case.

Even for people conversant with computational skills, and even given a wider exposure to such skills, there are still problems. Computation can be a tedious business, and does not necessarily have a transparent semantics for the problems (particularly in psychology) that we may try to address. Even if it does, computation does not of itself solve the substantive problems. These as always require the creativity and insight of the individual; however much computation may facilitate their expression and their exploration. Current computational metaphors may be much more apposite than those of the reflex machine. But still in undertaking further explorations, problems remain of someone, a person, conceiving processes which could undertake activities of mind. Then there is the problem of sharing whatever insights are gained: other people's computer programs are notoriously difficult to understand.

However, the advent of computation seems at least to have brought with it one possibility for the resolving the apparent contradiction of the polar extremes of mechanism on one hand (for the computer is entirely mechanical) and personal experience on the other (for to write or understand a computer program can be a matter of creative personal experience).

Just as Lashley in his writings constantly sought some rapprochement between the mechanical stuff of the brain and the issue of consciousness, the neural pathway, and the perceiver's independence of it, so I have tried to show that with the new metaphors of computational cognition, these searchings can be carried forward a little. Around the idea of the 'effort after meaning' emerges a synthesis. It is not just a restatement of the different categories that are mechanism and experience, not just a distinction between them, not just a juxtaposition. Rather it can be seen as an invitation to create a new mode of psychological theory. Just as the contradictions which arise between aspiration and execution of a LOGO program (bugs) are an invitation to create a better theory, so the apparent contradiction between the mechanism of the brain and the experience of being a person with this particular piece of mechanism invites a better theory. It seems possible that this contradiction is beginning to be resolved within a growing theory of meaning, representation and cognitive schemata.

Bibliography

AARONSON, L.R. (1956) Further studies on orientation and jumping behaviour in the goby fish *bathygobius soporator*. *Anatomical Record* 125, 606.

ABELSON, R.P. (1973) Simulation of belief systems. In R.C. Schank and K.M. Colby (eds) *Computer Models of Thought and Language*. San Francisco: W.H. Freeman.

ABERCROMBIE, M.L.J. (1960) *The Anatomy of Judgement*. London: Hutchinson.

ADRIAN, E.D. (1928) *The Basis of Sensation*. London: Christophers.

BADDELEY, A. and WARRINGTON, E. (1970) Amnesia and the distinction between long- and short-term memory. *Journal of Verbal Learning and Verbal Behaviour* 9, 176-89.

BARD, P. (1940) The hypothalamus and sexual behaviour. *Publications of the Association for Research on Nervous and Mental Disease* 20, 551-79.

BARLOW, H.B. (1961) Possible principles underlying the transformation of sensory messages. In W.A. Rosenblith (ed.) *Sensory Communication*. Cambridge, Mass.: M.I.T. Press.

BARLOW, H.B. (1975) Visual experience and cortical development. *Nature* 258, 199-204.

BARLOW, H.B., BLAKEMORE, C. and PETTIGREW, J.D. (1967) The neural mechanism of binocular depth perception. *Journal of physiology* 193, 327-42.

BARLOW, H.B., FITZHUGH, R. and KUFFLER, S.W. (1953) Change of organization in the receptive fields of the cat's retina during dark adaptation. *Journal of Physiology* 137, 338-54.

BARLOW, H.B. and HILL, R.M. (1963) Selective sensitivity to direction of movement in ganglion cells of rabbit retina. *Science* 139, 412-14.

BARTHES, R. (1972) *Mythologies*. London: Jonathan Cape.

BARTLETT, F.C. (1932) *Remembering*. Cambridge: Cambridge University press.

BEKESY, G. von (1967) *Sensory Inhibition*. Princeton: Princeton University press.

BERNARD, C. (1865) *Introduction à l'étude de la médicine experimentale*. Paris:

BITTERMAN, M.E. (1965) The evolution of intelligence. *Scientific American* 212, 92-100.

BLAKEMORE, C. and CAMPBELL, F.W. (1969) On the existence of neurones in the human visual system selectively sensitive to the orientation and size of retinal image. *Journal of Physiology* 203, 237-60.

BLAKEMORE, C. and TOBIN, E.A. (1972) Lateral inhibition between orientation detectors in the cat's visual cortex. *Experimental Brain Research* 15, 439-40.

BOBROW, D.G. (1970) Natural language interaction systems. In S. Kaneff (ed.) *Picture Language Machines*. London: Academic Press.

BOOTH, D.A. (1970) Neurochemical changes correlated with learning and memory retention. In G. Ungar (ed.) *Molecular Mechanisms in Memory and Learning*. New York: Plenum.

BRANSFORD, J. and FRANKS, J. (1971) Abstraction of linguistic ideas. *Cognitive Psychology* 2, 331-50.

BRESLER, D.E. and BITTERMAN, M.E. (1969) Learning in fish with transplanted brain tissue. *Science* 163, 590-2.

BURNS, B.D. (1958) *The Mammalian Cerebral Cortex*. London: Arnold.

BURNS, B.D. (1968) *The Uncertain Nervous System*. London: Arnold.

CAMPBELL, F.W., CLELAND, B.G., COOPER, G.F. and ENROTH-CUGELL, C. (1968) The angular selectivity of visual cortical cells to moving gratings. *Journal of Physiology* 198, 237-50.

CAMPBELL, F.W., COOPER, G.F. and ENROTH-CUGELL, C. (1969) The spatial selectivity of the visual cells of the cat. *Journal of physiology* 203, 223-35.

CAMPBELL, F. and GREEN, D.G. (1965) Optical and retinal factors affecting visual resolution. *Journal of Physiology* 181, 576-93.

CAMPBELL, F. and ROBSON, J.G. (1968) Application of Fourier analysis to the visibility of gratings. *Journal of Physiology* 197, 551-66.

CHOMSKY, N. (1965) *Aspects of the Theory of Syntax*. Cambridge, Mass.: M.I.T. Press.

CHOMSKY, N. (1968) *Language and Mind*. New York: Harcourt, Brace and World.

CHOMSKY, N. and HAMPSHIRE, S. (1968) The Study of Language. *The Listener* 79, 687-91.

CLOWES, M. (1971) On seeing things. *Artificial Intelligence* 2, 79-116.

CLOWES, M.B. (1973) Artificial intelligence and psychology. A.I.S.B. Bulletin No. 1.

CLOWES, M.B. (1973) Man the creative machine: a perspective from artificial intelligence research. In E.J. Benthall (ed.) *The Limits of Human Nature*. London: Allen Lane.

CLOWES, M.B. (1973) From A.I.S.B. Summer School, *cit.* Weir, S. (1975) The perception of motion: actions motives and feelings. Edinburgh University: Department of Artificial Intelligence Research Report No. 13.

CORNSWEET, T. (1970) *Visual Perception*. London: Academic Press.

COWAN, J.D. (1972) Stochastic models of neuroelectric activity. In C.H. Waddington (ed.) *Towards a Theoretical Biology, Vol. IV*. Edinburgh: Edinburgh University Press.

CRAIK, K. (1943) *The Nature of Explanation*. Cambridge: Cambridge University Press.

DESCARTES, R. (1664) *L'homme*. Originally published in Paris. Selections translated by E. Clarke and C. O'Malley (1968) *The Human Brain and Spinal Cord*. Berkeley: University of California Press.

DESCARTES, R. (1667) Méditations métaphysique. Originally published in Paris. Selections translated by E. Clarke and C. O'Malley (1968) *The Human Brain and Spinal Cord*. Berkeley: University of California Press.

DEUTSCH, J.A. (1971) The cholinergic synapse and the site of memory. *Science* 174, 788-94.

DUNCKER, K. (1945) On problem solving. (Translated by L.S. Lees.) *Psychological Monograph* 58, No. 270.

FALK, G. (1972) Interpretation of imperfect line data as a 3-dimensional scene. *Artificial Intelligence* 3, 101-44.

FITZSIMONS, J.T. (1963) The effect of slow infusions of hypertonic solutions on drinking and drinking thresholds in rats. *Journal of Physiology* 167, 344-54.

FLOURENS, M.J.P. (1824) *Recherches expérimentales sur les propriétés, et les jonctions du système nerveau dans les animaux vertébrés*. Paris: Crevot.

GENNERY, D.B. (1973) Determination of optical transfer function by inspection of frequency domain plot. *Journal of the Optical Society of America* 63, 1571-7.

GEORGESON, M.A. and SULLIVAN, G.D. (1975) Contrast constancy: deblurring in human vision by spatial frequency channels. *Journal of Physiology* 252, 627-56.

GIBSON, J.J. (1966) *The Senses Considered as Perceptual Systems*. Boston: Houghton.

GINSBERG, A.P. (1975) Is the illusory triangle physical or imaginary? *Nature* 257, 219-20.

GIRDEN, E., METTLER, F.A., FINCH, G. and CULLER, E. (1930) Conditioned responses in a decorticate dog to acoustic, thermal and tactile stimulation. *Journal of Comparative Psychology* 21, 367-85.

GOFFMAN, E. (1974) *Frame Analysis*. New York: Harper and Row.

GOLDSTEIN, I.P. (1974) Understanding simple picture programs. Artificial Intelligence and the Simulation of Behaviour Conference, University of Sussex.

GOMBRICH, E.H. (1960) *Art and Illusion*. London: Phaidon.

GONZALEZ, R.L., ROBERTS, W.A. and BITTERMAN, M.E. (1964) Learning in adult rats with extensive lesions made in infancy. *American Journal of Psychology* 77, 547-62.

GOODWIN, B.C. (1976) *Analytical Physiology of Cells and Developing Organisms*. London: Academic Press.

GREENSPOON, J. (1955) The reinforcing effect of two spoken sounds on the frequencies of two responses. *American Journal of Psychology* 68, 409-16.

GREGORY, R.L. (1961) The brain as an engineering problem. In W.H. Thorpe and O.L. Zangwill (eds) *Current Problems in Animal Behaviour*. Cambridge: Cambridge University Press.

GREGORY, R.L. (1970) *The Intelligent Eye*. London: Weidenfeld and Nicolson.

GREGORY, R.L. (1973) The confounded eye. In R.L. Gregory and E.H. Gombrich (eds) *Illusion in Nature and Art*. London: Duckworth.

GRINDLEY, G.C. (1927) The neural basis of purposive activity. *British Journal of Psychology* 18, 168-88.

GRINDLEY, G.C. (1932) The formation of a simple habit in guinea pigs. *British Journal of Psychology* 23, 127-47.

GROSS, C.G., ROSHA-MIRANDA, C.E. and BENDER, D.B. (1972) Visual properties of neurons in inferotemporal cortex of the macaque. *Journal of Neurophysiology* 35, 96-111.

GUZMAN, A. (1969) Decomposition of a visual scene into three-dimensional bodies. In A. Grasselli (ed.) *Automatic Interpretation and Classification of Images*. London: Academic Press.

HAGSTROM, W.O. (1965) *The Scientific Community*. New York: Basic Books.

HAMILTON, E. and CAIRNS, H. (1961) *The Collected Dialogues of Plato*. Princeton: Princeton University Press.

HEAD, H. (1920) *Studies in Neurology*. Oxford: Oxford University Press.

HEBB, D.O. (1949) *The Organization of Behaviour*. New York: Wiley.

HEBB, D.O. (1963) Introduction to K.S. Lashley *Brain Mechanisms and Intelligence*. New York: Dover.

HEIDER, F. and SIMMEL, M. (1944) An experimental study of apparent behaviour. *American Journal of Psychology* 57, 243-59.

HELMHOLTZ, H. von (1860) *Treatise on physiological optics, Vol. II*. Edited by J.P.C. Southall (1962). New York: Dover.

HELMHOLTZ, H. von (1862) *On the Sensations of Tone*. English translation (1954). New York: Dover.

HELMHOLTZ, H. von (1866) *Treatise on physiological optics, Vol. III*. Edited by J.P.C. Southall (1962). New York: Dover.

HERING, E. (1878) *Zur Lehre vom Lichtsinne*. Berlin.

HETHERINGTON, A.W. and RANSON, S.W. (1940) Hypothalamic lesions and adiposity in the rat. *Anatomical Record* 78, 149-72.

HEWITT, C. (1971) Procedural embedding of knowledge in PLANNER. *International Joint Conference on Artificial Intelligence*, 1971. London.

HICK, W.E. (1952) On the rate of gain of information. *Quarterly Journal of Experimental Psychology* 4, 11-26.

HIRSCH, H.V.B. (1972) Visual perception in cats after environmental surgery. *Experimental Brain Research* 15, 405-23.

HIRSCH, H.V.B. and SPINELLI, D.N. (1970) Visual experience modifies distribution of horizontally and vertically oriented receptive fields in cats. *Science* 168, 869-71.

HODOS, W. (1970) Evolutionary interpretation of neural and behavioural studies in living vertebrates. In F.O. Schmitt (ed.) *The Neurosciences: Second Study Program*. New York: Rockefeller University Press.

HOLT, J. (1969) *How Children Fail*. London: Pelican.

HORN, G. and HILL, R.M. (1964) Habituation of the response to sensory stimuli of neurones in the brain stem of rabbits. *Nature* 202, 296-8.

HORRIDGE, G.A. (1965) The electrophysiological approach to learning in isolatable ganglia. *Animal Behaviour Supplement* 1, 163-82.

HORRIDGE, G.A. (1968) *Interneurons*. San Francisco: W.H. Freeman.

HORRIDGE, G.A. (1969) The interpretation of behaviour in terms of interneurons. In M.A.B. Brazier (ed.) *The Interneuron*. Berkeley: University of California Press.

HORRIDGE, G.A. (1973) Integration in nervous systems. In E.C. Carterette and M.P. Friedman (eds) *Handbook of Perception, Vol. III*. New York: Academic Press.

HUBEL, D.H. and WIESEL, T.N. (1959) Receptive fields and single neurones in the cat's striate cortex. *Journal of Physiology* 148, 574-91.

HUBEL, D.H. and WIESEL, T.N. (1962) Receptive fields, binocular interaction and functional architecture in the cat's visual cortex. *Journal of Physiology* 160, 106-54.

HUBEL, D.H. and WIESEL, T.N. (1965) Receptive fields and functional architecture in two nonstriate visual areas (18 and 19) of the cat. *Journal of Neurophysiology* 28, 229-89.

HUFFMAN, D. (1971) Impossible objects as nonsense sentences. In B. Meltzer and D. Michie (eds) *Machine Intelligence 6*. Edinburgh: Edinburgh University Press.

HUGHLINGS-JACKSON, J. (1959) *Selected Writings of John Hughlings-Jackson*. Edited by J. Taylor. New York: Basic Books.

HULL, C.L. (1951) *Essentials of Behaviour*. New Haven: Yale University Press.

HUYGENS, C. (1665) Sympathie des horloges. In Société Hollandaise des Sciences (eds) *Oeuvres complètes de Christian Huygens, Vol. 17*. La Haye: Nijhoff.

IKEDA, H. and WRIGHT, M.J. (1974) Evidence for 'sustained' and 'transient' neurones in the cat's visual cortex. *Vision Research* 14, 133-6.

JERISON, H.J. (1973) *Evolution of the Brain and Intelligence*. New York: Academic Press.

JOHANSSON, G. (1971) Visual motion perception: a model for visual motion and space perception from changing proximal stimulations. University of Uppsala, Department of Psychology, Report 98.

JOHN, E.R. (1967) *Mechanisms of Memory*. New York: Academic Press.

JOUVET, M. (1967) Neurophysiology of the states of sleep. *Physiological Reviews* 47, 117-77.

KANDEL, E.R. (1974) An invertebrate system for the cellular analysis of simple behaviors and their modification. In F.O. Schmitt and F.G. Worden (eds) *The Neurosciences: Third Study Program*. Cambridge, Mass: M.I.T. Press.

KASAMATSU, A. and HIRAI, T. (1966) An electrencephalographic study on the Zen meditation (zazen). *Folio Psychiatrica and Neurologica Japonica* 20, 315-36.

KELLY, G.A. (1955) *The Psychology of Personal Constructs*. New York: Norton.

KENT, E. and GROSSMAN, S.P. (1970) Evidence for a conflict interpretation of anomalous effects of rewarding brain stimulation. *Journal of Comparative and Physiological Psychology* 69, 381-90.

KERKUT, G.A., OLIVER, G., RICK, J.J. and WALKER, R.J. (1970) Biochemical changes during learning in an insect ganglion. *Nature* 227, 722-3.

KIMBLE, G. (1961) *Hilgard and Marquis's Conditioning and Learning*. London: Methuen.

KUHN, T.S. (1957) *The Copernican Revolution*. Cambridge, Mass: Harvard University Press.

KUHN, T.S. (1962) *The Structure of Scientific Revolutions*. Chicago: Chicago University Press.

LAING, R.D. (1967) *The Politics of Experience*. London: Penguin.

LAKATOS, I. (1970) Falsification and the methodology of scientific research programmes. In I. Lakatos, and A. Musgrave (eds) *Criticism and the Growth of Knowledge*. Cambridge: Cambridge University Press.

LASHLEY, K.S. (1929) *Brain Mechanisms and Intelligence*. Chicago: University of Chicago Press.

LASHLEY, K.S. (1930) Basic neural mechanisms in behaviour. *Psychological Review* 37, 1-24.

LASHLEY, K.S. (1938) The mechanism of vision. XV. Preliminary studies of the rat's capacity for detail vision. *Journal of General Physiology* 18, 123-93.

LASHLEY, K.S. (1938) An experimental analysis of instinctive behaviour. *Psychological Review,* 45, 445-471.

LASHLEY, K.S. (1942) The problem of cerebral organization in vision. *Biological Symposia* 7, 301-22.

LASHLEY, K.S. (1949) Persistent problems in the evolution of mind. *Quarterly Review of Biology* 24, 28-42.

LASHLEY, K.S. (1950) In search of the engram. *Symposia of the Society of Experimental Biology* 4, 454-82.

LASHLEY, K.S. (1951) The problem of serial order in behaviour. In L.A. Jeffress (ed.) *Cerebral Mechanisms in Behaviour*. New York: Wiley.

LASHLEY, K.S. (1951) Discussion at 'Symposium on the Brain and the Mind', American Neurological Association, *cit.* S. Cobb A salute from neurologists. In F.A. Beach, D.O. Hebb, C.T. Morgan and H.W. Nissen (eds) (1960) *The Neuropsychology of Lashley*. New York: McGraw-Hill.

LASHLEY, K.S. (1957) Letter cited by S. Cobb (1960) A salute from neurologists. In F.A. Beach, D.O. Hebb, C.T. Morgan and H.W. Nissen (eds) *The Neuropsychology of Lashley*. New York: McGraw-Hill.

LASHLEY, K.S. and McCARTHY, D.A. (1926) The survival of the maze habit after cerebellar injuries. *Journal of Comparative Psychology* 6, 428-33.

LEONARD, J. (1959) Tactual choice reactions 1. *Quarterly Journal of Experimental Psychology* 11, 76-83.

LETTVIN, J.Y., MATTURANA, H.R., McCULLOCH, W.S. and PITTS, W.H. (1959) What the frog's eye tells the frog's brain. *Proceedings of the Institute of Radio Engineers* 47, 1940-1951.

LINDSAY, P.H. and NORMAN, D.A. (1972) *Human Information Processing*. New York: Academic Press.

LORENTE de NO, R. (1933) Studies on the structure of the cerebral cortex. *Journal für Psychologie and Neurologie* 45, 381-438.

LORENZ, K. (1969) Innate bases of learning. In K.H. Pribram (ed.) *On the Biology of Learning*. New York: Harcourt Brace and World.

LURIA, A.R. (1970) The functional organization of the brain. *Scientific American* 222, 66-78.

McCULLOCH, W. and PITTS, W. (1943) A logical calculus of the ideas immanent in nervous activity. *Bulletin of Mathematical Biophysics* 5, 115.

MACKINTOSH, N.J. (1976) Conditioning as the perception of causal relations. In R. Butts and J. Hintikka (eds) *Proceedings of the 5th International Congress of Logic. Methodology and Philosophy of Science.* London, Ontario: University of Western Ontario Press.

McLEOD, I.D.G. and ROSENFELD, A. (1974) The visibility of gratings: spatial frequency channels or bar-detecting units. *Vision Research* 14, 909-15.

MACKWORTH, A. (1976) Model driven interpretation in intelligent vision systems. *Perception* 5, 347-70.

MARCEL, A.J. (1970) Some constraints on sequential and parallel processing and the limits of attention. In A.F. Saunders (ed.) *Attention and Performance III*. Amsterdam: North-Holland Publishing.

MARR, D. (1975) Analysing natural images: a computational theory of texture vision. M.I.T. AI Memo 334.
MARR, D. (1976) Early processing of visual information. *Philosophical Transactions of the Royal Society of London*, Series B.275, 483-519.
MATTHEWS, G.V.T. (1955) *Bird Navigation*. Cambridge: Cambridge University Press.
MAXWELL, J.C. (1868) On governors. *Proceedings of the Royal Society* 16, 270-83.
MAYHEW, J.E.W., and ANSTIS, S.M. (1972) Movement after-effects contingent on colour intensity and pattern. *Perception and Psychophysics* 12, 77-85.
MECH, L.D. (1971) *The Wolf: The Ecology and Behaviour of an Endangered Species*. Garden City, N.Y.: Doubleday.
MERTON, R.K. (1942) The institutional imperatives of science. Reprinted in R.K. Merton (1967) *Social Theory and Social Structure*. Glencoe: Free Press.
MICHOTTE, A. (1963) *The Perception of Causality*. London: Methuen.
MILGRAM, S. (1974) *Obedience to Authority: An Experimental View*. London: Tavistock.
MILLER, N.E. (1971) *Selected Papers*. Chicago: Aldine Publishing.
MILNER, B. (1974) Hemispheric specialization: scope and limits. In F.O. Schmitt and F.G. Worden (eds) *The Neurosciences: Third Study Program*. Cambridge, Mass.: M.I.T. Press.
MINSKY, M. (1977) Frame system theory. In P.N. Johnson-Laird and P. Wason (eds) *Thinking: Readings in Cognitive Science*. Cambridge: Cambridge University Press.
MITCHELL, D.E., FREEMAN, R.D., MILLDOT, M. and HAEGERSTROM, G. (1973) Meridional amblyopia: evidence for modification of the human visual system by early visual experience. *Vision Research* 13, 535-58.
MOWBRAY, G. and RHOADES, M. (1959) On the reduction of choice reaction times with practice. *Quarterly Journal of Experimental Psychology* 11, 16-23.
NEISSER, U. (1964) Visual search. *Scientific American* 210, 94-102.
NEISSER, U. (1967) *Cognitive Psychology*. New York: Appleton-Century.
OATLEY, K. (1970) Brain mechanisms and motivation. *Nature* 255, 797-801.
OATLEY, K. (1972) *Brain Mechanisms and Mind*. London: Thames and Hudson.
OATLEY, K. (1973) Simulation and theory of thirst. In A.N. Epstein, H.R. Kissileff and E. Stellar (eds) *The Neuropsychology of Thirst: New Findings and Advances in Concepts*. Washington, DC: V.H. Winston.
OATLEY, K. (1974) Circadian rhythms and representations of the environment in motivational systems. In D.J. McFarland (ed.) *Motivational Control Systems Analysis*. London: Academic Press.
OATLEY, K. (1974) Mental maps for navigation. *New Scientist* 64, 863-6.
OATLEY, K. (1975) Clock mechanisms of sleep. *New Scientist* 66, 371-4.
OATLEY, K. (1976) Why isn't the world more fuzzy than it is? *New Scientist* 71, 338-40.
OATLEY, K. and GOODWIN, B.C. (1971) The explanation and

investigation of biological rhythms. In W.P. Colquhoun (ed.) *Biological Rhythms and Human Performance*. London: Academic Press.

OATLEY, K. and TOATES, F.M. (1971) Frequency analysis of the thirst control system. *Nature* 232, 562-4.

O'BRIEN, V. (1958) Contour perception, illusion and reality. *Journal of the Optical Society of America* 48, 112-19.

OLDS, J. and MILNER, P. (1954) Positive reinforcement produced by electrical stimulation of septal area and other regions of rat brain. *Journal of Comparative and Physiological Psychology* 47, 419-27.

OYSTER, C.W. (1968) The analysis of image motion by the rabbit retina. *Journal of Physiology* 199, 613-35.

PAPERT, S. (1973) Uses of technology to enhance education. M.I.T. AI Memo 298.

PAVLOV, I.P. (1927) *Conditioned Reflexes*. Oxford: Oxford University Press.

PENFIELD, W. and RASMUSSEN, T. (1950) *The Cerebral Cortex of Man*. New York: Macmillan.

POLLEN, D.A. and TAYLOR, J.H. (1974) The striate cortex and the spatial analysis of visual space. In F.O. Schmitt and F.G. Worden (eds) *The Neurosciences: Third Study Program*. Cambridge, Mass: M.I.T. Press.

POLYA, G. (1945) *How to Solve It*. Princeton, N.J.: Princeton University Press.

POPPER, K.R. (1963) *Conjectures and Refutations*. London: Routledge and Kegan Paul.

PORTER, P.B. (1954) Another puzzle picture. *American Journal of Psychology* 67, 550-51.

PREMACK, D. (1971) Language in chimpanzee? *Science* 172, 808-22.

RAPHAEL, B. (1976) *The Thinking Computer: Mind inside Matter*. San Francisco: W.H. Freeman.

RATLIFF, F. (1965) *Mach Bands: Quantative Studies on Neural Networks in the Retina*. San Francisco: Holden-Day.

RATLIFF, F. and HARTLINE, H.K. (1974) *Studies of Excitation and Inhibition in the Retina*. London: Chapman and Hall.

RAZRAN, G.H.S. (1938) Music, art and the conditioned response. Paper read at the Eastern Psychological Association. Quoted by Verhave *op. cit.*

RESCORLA, R.A. and WAGNER, A.R. (1972) A theory of Pavlovian conditioning variation in the effectiveness of reinforcement and non-reinforcement. In A.H. Black and W.F. Prokasy (eds) *Classical Conditioning II. Current Research and Theory*. New York: Appleton-Century-Crofts.

ROBERTS, L.G. (1965) Machine perception of three-dimensional solids. I.J.T. Tippett *et al* (eds) *Optical and Electro-optical Information Processing*. Cambridge, Mass.: M.I.T. Press.

ROEDER, K.D. (1966) Auditory system of noctuid moths. *Science* 154, 1515-21.

ROSE, S.P.R. (1973) *The Conscious Brain*. London: Weidenfeld and Nicolson.

ROSENZWEIG, M.R. (1970) Evidence for anatomical and chemical changes in the brain during primary learning. In K.H. Pribram and D.E.

D.E. Broadbent (eds) *Biology of Memory*. London: Academic Press.
ROSENZWEIG, M.R., BENNETT, E.L. and DIAMOND, M.C. (1972) Brain changes in response to experience. *Scientific American* 226, 22-9.
ROSS, D.M. (1965) The behaviour of sessile coelenterates in relation to some conditioning experiments. *Animal Behaviour Supplement 1* 13, 43-52.
SCHNEIDER, G.C. (1969) Two visual systems. *Science* 163, 891-5.
SCHWEDER, R.A. (1977) Likeness and likelihood in everyday thought: magical thinking and everyday judgements about personality. *Current Anthropology* (in press).
SHALLICE, T. and WARRINGTON, E. (1970) Independent functioning of verbal memory stores: a neurophysiological study. *Quarterly Journal of Experimental Psychology* 22, 261-73.
SHEPARD, R.N. and METZLER, J. (1971) Mental rotation of three-dimensional objects. *Science* 171, 701-3.
SHERRINGTON, C.S. (1906) *The Integrative Action of the Nervous System*. New Haven: Yale University Press.
SHIRAI, Y. (1975) Analysing intensity arrays using knowledge about scenes. In P. Winston (ed.) *The Psychology of Computer Vision*. New York: McGraw-Hill.
SHOLL, D.A. (1956) *The Organisation of the Cerebral Cortex*. London: Methuen.
SIMPSON, P.J. (1972) High speed memory scanning: stability and generality. *Journal of Experimental Psychology* 96, 239-46.
SKINNER, B.F. (1938) *The Behaviour of Organisms*. New York: Appleton-Century-Crofts.
SKINNER, B.F. (1972) *Beyond Freedom and Dignity*. London: Cape.
SMITH, S. (1957) *Not Waving but Drowning*. London: Andre Deutsch.
SPENCER, H. (1899) *Principles of Psychology* (3rd edition). New York: Appleton.
SPENCER, W.A., THOMPSON, R.F. and NIELSON, D.R. (1966) Response decrement of flexion reflex in acute spinal cat and transient restoration by strong stimuli. *Journal of Neurophysiology* 29, 221-39.
SPERRY, R.W. (1967) Split brain approach to learning problems. In G.C. Quarton, T. Melmechuk and F.O. Schmitt (eds) *The Neurosciences: First Study Program*. New York: Rockefeller University Press.
SPERRY, R.W. (1974) Lateral specialization in the surgically separated hemispheres. In F.O. Schmitt and F.G. Worden (eds) *The Neurosciences: Third Study Program*. Cambridge, Mass.: M.I.T. Press.
STARK, L. and SHERMAN, P.M. (1957) A servoanalytic study of the consensual pupil reflex. *Journal of Neurophysiology* 20, 17-26.
STERNBERG, S. (1969) Memory scanning: mental processes revealed by reaction time experiments. *American Scientist* 57, 421-57.
STERNBERG, S. (1975) Memory scanning: new findings and current controversies. *Quarterly Journal of Experimental Psychology* 27, 1-32.
STEVENS, S.S. (1961) To honour Fechner and repeal his law. *Science* 133, 80-6.
STONE, J. and DREHER, B. (1973) Projection of X- and Y-cells of the cat's lateral geniculate nucleus to areas 17 and 18 of visual cortex. *Journal of Neurophysiology* 36, 551-67.

SULLIVAN, G.D., GEORGESON, M.A. and OATLEY, K. (1972) Channels for spatial frequency selection and the detection of single bars by the human visual system. *Vision Research* 12, 383-94.

SUTHERLAND, N.S. (1961) Figural after-effects and apparent size. *Quarterly Journal of Experimental Psychology* 13, 222-8.

SUTHERLAND, N.S. (1970) Is the brain a physical system? In R. Borger and F. Cioffi (eds) *Explanations in the Behavioural Sciences*. Cambridge: Cambridge University Press.

SUTHERLAND, N.S. (1973) Intelligent picture processing. Paper presented at the Conference on the Evolution of the Nervous System and Behavior, Florida State University, 1973.

SUTHERLAND, N.S. (1975) Review of *Animal Nature and Human Nature* by W.H. Thorpe. *Nature* 254, 219-20.

TEITELBAUM, P. (1967) *Physiological Psychology: Fundamental Principles*. Englewood Cliffs, N.J.: Prentice-Hall.

TEITELBAUM, P. (1967) The biology of drive. In G.C. Quarton, T. Melnechuck, and F.O. Schmitt (eds) *The Neurosciences: First Study Program*. New York: Rockefeller University Press.

THOMPSON, R.F. (1967) *Foundations of Physiological Psychology*. New York: Harper and Row.

THOMPSON, R. and McCONNELL, J. (1955) Classical conditioning in the planarian *dugesia dorotocephala*. *Journal of Comparative and Physiological Psychology* 48, 65-8.

THORNDIKE, E.L. (1911) *Animal Intelligence*. New York: Macmillan.

THORPE, W.H. (1975) *Animal Nature and Human Nature*. London: Methuen.

TINBERGEN, N. (1951) *The Study of Instinct*. Oxford: Oxford University Press.

TOATES, F.M. and OATLEY, K. (1970) Computer simulation of thirst and water balance. *Medical and Biological Engineering* 8, 71-87.

TROWELL, J.A., PANKSEPP, J. and GANDALMAN, R. (1969) An incentive model of rewarding brain stimulation. *Psychological Review* 76, 264-81.

TULVING, E. and MADIGAN, S.A. (1972) Memory and verbal learning. *Annual Review of Psychology* 21, 437-84.

TURING, A.M. (1936) On computable numbers, with an application to the Entscheidungs problem. *Proceedings of the London Mathematical Society*, Series 2 42, 230-65.

TURING, A.M. (1950) Computing machinery and intelligence. *Mind* 59, 433-60.

UEXKÜLL, J. von (1934) Stroll through the worlds of animals and man. Translated in C.H. Schiller (ed.) (1957) *Instinctive Behaviour*. London: Methuen.

UPDYKE, B.V. (1974) Characteristics of unit responses in superior colliculus of *Cebus* monkey. *Journal of Neurophysiology* 37, 896-909.

UTTAL, W.R. (1973) The Psychobiology of Sensory Coding. New York: Harper and Row.

VALENSTEIN, E.S. (1973) *Brain Control*. New York: Wiley.

VANDERWOLF, C.H. (1971) Limbic diencephalic mechanisms of voluntary movement. *Psychological Review* 78, 83-113.

VERHAVE, T. (1966) An introduction to the experimental analysis of behaviour. In T. Verhave (ed.) *The Experimental Analysis of Behaviour: Selected Readings*. New York: Appleton-Century-Crofts.

WALTER, W.G., COOPER, R., ALDRIDGE, V.J. and WINTER, A.L. (1964) Contingent negative variation: an electric sign of sensori-motor association and expectancy in the human brain. *Nature* 203, 380-4.

WALTZ, D. (1975) Understanding line drawings of scenes with shadows. In P. Winston (ed.) *The Psychology of Computer Vision*. New York: McGraw-Hill.

WEINER, N. (1958) *Cybernetics*. New York: Wiley.

WEIR, S. (1975) The perception of motion: actions, motives and feelings. In Progress in Perception. University of Edinburgh, Department of Artificial Intelligence Report No. 13.

WEISS, P. (1967) One plus one does not equal two. In G.C. Quarton, T. Melnechuk and F.O. Schmitt (eds) *The Neurosciences: First Study Program*. New York: Rockefeller University Press.

WEIZENBAUM, J. (1965) ELIZA — A computer program for the study of natural language communication between man and machine. *Communications of the Association for Computing Machinery* 9, 36-45.

WEIZENBAUM, J. (1976) *Computer Power and Human Reason*. San Francisco: W.H. Freeman.

WERBLIN, F.S. and DOWLING, J.E. (1969) Organization of the retina of the mud puppy: II Intracellular recording. *Journal of Neurophysiology* 32, 339-55.

WERTHEIMER, M. (1969) *Productive Thinking*. (Enlarged edition) London: Tavistock Publications.

WINOGRAD, T. (1971) Procedures as a representation for data in a computer program for understanding natural language. M.I.T. AI Memo TR 17.

WINSTON, P.H. (1972) The MIT Robot. In B. Meltzer and D. Michie (eds) *Machine Intelligence 7*. Edinburgh: Edinburgh University Press.

WINSTON, P.H. (1975) *The Psychology of Computer Vision*. New York: McGraw-Hill.

WITTGENSTEIN, L. (1953) *Philosophical Investigations*. Translated by G.E.M. Anscombe (1968). Oxford: Blackwell.

YATES, F.A. (1964) *Giordano Bruno and the Hermetic Tradition*. London: Routledge and Kegan Paul.

YATES, F.A. (1966) *The Art of Memory*. London: Routledge and Kegan Paul.

ZANGWILL, O.L. (1961) Lashley's concept of cerebral mass action. In W.H. Thorpe and O.L. Zangwill (eds) *Current Problems in Animal Behaviour*. Cambridge: Cambridge University Press.

Index